CONTENTS

Chapter 1: Introduction   1
Chapter 2: Anatomy of Carotid Arteries   4
Chapter 3: Atherosclerosis and Carotid Artery Stenosis   20
Chapter 4: Diagnosis and Imaging Techniques   43
Chapter 5: Grading and Classification   63
Chapter 6: Natural History of Carotid Artery Stenosis   75
Chapter 7: Medical Management   90
Chapter 8: Surgical Interventions   113
Chapter 9: Novel Therapeutic Approaches   127
Chapter 10: Post-Treatment Care and Follow-up   140
Chapter 11: Integrative and Holistic Approaches   155

CHAPTER 1: INTRODUCTION

Definition of Carotid Artery Disease

Carotid Artery Disease (CAD), also known as Carotid Artery Stenosis, is a vascular condition characterized by the narrowing or blockage of the carotid arteries, major blood vessels located in the neck that supply blood to the brain. The primary cause of carotid artery disease is atherosclerosis, a process where fatty deposits, cholesterol, and other substances build up on the inner walls of the arteries, forming plaques. As these plaques accumulate, they can reduce blood flow to the brain, leading to serious health complications such as stroke or transient ischemic attack (TIA).

The severity of carotid artery disease is often assessed based on the degree of stenosis, which refers to the percentage of narrowing in the carotid arteries. Stenosis greater than 70% is generally considered significant and may warrant intervention to prevent adverse outcomes.

Historical Perspective

The historical understanding of carotid artery disease dates back centuries, with early observations and theories laying the groundwork for contemporary knowledge. In the 19th century, physicians began recognizing the association between arterial diseases and strokes. However, it wasn't until the mid-20th century that advancements in medical imaging and diagnostic techniques allowed for a more detailed understanding of the anatomy and pathology of the carotid arteries.

The landmark North American Symptomatic Carotid Endarterectomy Trial (NASCET) and the European Carotid Surgery Trial (ECST) conducted in the 1980s and 1990s played a pivotal role in shaping our understanding of carotid artery disease. These trials provided crucial insights into the natural history of the disease, optimal management strategies, and contributed to the development of standardized criteria for grading and classifying carotid artery stenosis.

Epidemiology and Prevalence

Epidemiological studies have shed light on the global burden of carotid artery disease, emphasizing its significance in public health. The prevalence of carotid artery stenosis increases with age, and it is more common in males than females. Lifestyle factors, such as smoking, hypertension, diabetes, and high cholesterol, contribute significantly to the development and progression of the disease.

Geographical variations exist, with higher rates reported in regions where these risk factors are more prevalent. Additionally, there is a notable association between carotid artery disease and other cardiovascular conditions, reinforcing the interconnected nature of vascular health.

Risk Factors

Understanding the risk factors associated with carotid artery disease is crucial for preventive measures and targeted interventions. Several modifiable and non-modifiable risk factors contribute to the development and progression of CAD.

Modifiable Risk Factors:

- **Smoking:** Tobacco smoke contains harmful substances

that accelerate atherosclerosis and increase the risk of plaque formation.
- **Hypertension:** Elevated blood pressure places additional stress on the arterial walls, promoting the development of plaques.
- **Dyslipidemia:** Abnormal levels of cholesterol and lipids contribute to the formation of atherosclerotic plaques.
- **Diabetes:** Individuals with diabetes are at higher risk due to the impact of insulin resistance on vascular health.
- **Obesity:** Excess body weight is linked to various risk factors, including diabetes and hypertension.

Non-Modifiable Risk Factors:

- **Age:** The risk of carotid artery disease increases with age, with the elderly being more susceptible.
- **Gender:** Men generally have a higher risk than women, although women's risk increases after menopause.
- **Genetics:** Family history of cardiovascular diseases can predispose individuals to carotid artery disease.

Addressing these risk factors through lifestyle modifications, medication, and regular monitoring is essential for preventing or managing carotid artery disease effectively. This multifaceted approach underscores the complexity of the disease and the need for personalized interventions based on individual risk profiles.

CHAPTER 2: ANATOMY OF CAROTID ARTERIES

Structure and Function of Carotid Arteries

The carotid arteries, paired vessels located on each side of the neck, are crucial components of the circulatory system responsible for supplying oxygenated blood to the brain. Understanding the intricate structure and function of these arteries is essential for comprehending the pathophysiology of carotid artery disease (CAD) and developing effective diagnostic and therapeutic strategies.

Structural Components:

The carotid arteries consist of three main layers: the intima, media, and adventitia.

1. **Intima:** The innermost layer, in direct contact with the blood flowing through the artery, is the intima. It is composed of a single layer of endothelial cells supported by a basement membrane. The endothelial cells play a pivotal role in maintaining vascular homeostasis, regulating blood flow, and preventing thrombosis.
2. **Media:** The middle layer, known as the media, is

primarily composed of smooth muscle cells embedded in an extracellular matrix containing elastin and collagen fibers. This layer provides structural support, elasticity, and contractility to the arterial walls. The smooth muscle cells regulate the diameter of the arteries in response to various physiological stimuli, ensuring appropriate blood flow to meet the brain's metabolic demands.
3. **Adventitia:** The outermost layer, the adventitia, is a connective tissue layer that anchors the artery to surrounding structures. It contains blood vessels, nerves, and collagen fibers, contributing to the overall strength and integrity of the arterial wall.

Functional Aspects:

The carotid arteries serve several critical functions, playing a key role in maintaining cerebral perfusion and overall brain health.

1. **Blood Supply to the Brain:** The primary function of the carotid arteries is to deliver oxygen and nutrients to the brain. Approximately 80% of the cerebral blood flow is derived from the carotid arteries, highlighting their significance in sustaining brain function.
2. **Regulation of Cerebral Blood Flow:** The smooth muscle cells within the arterial walls allow for dynamic regulation of blood flow to the brain. Autoregulatory mechanisms ensure a constant and appropriate supply of blood despite changes in systemic blood pressure.
3. **Baroreceptor Function:** The carotid arteries house baroreceptors, specialized sensory receptors that detect changes in blood pressure. These receptors relay information to the central nervous system, enabling rapid adjustments in vascular tone to maintain blood pressure within a narrow range.
4. **Carotid Sinus:** Located at the bifurcation of the common

carotid artery, the carotid sinus is a dilated region containing baroreceptors. It is particularly sensitive to changes in blood pressure and plays a crucial role in the reflex control of systemic vascular resistance.

Microscopic Anatomy:

Examining the microscopic anatomy of the carotid arteries provides insights into the cellular and molecular processes underlying their structure and function.

1. **Endothelial Cells:** The endothelial cells lining the intima form a continuous monolayer that serves as a semi-permeable barrier between the blood and the arterial wall. These cells actively participate in vascular homeostasis by releasing vasodilators (e.g., nitric oxide) and regulating the adhesion of blood cells.
2. **Smooth Muscle Cells:** The media is rich in smooth muscle cells, which contribute to the contractility and elasticity of the arteries. These cells respond to vasoactive substances, such as catecholamines, by modulating the vessel diameter to meet the dynamic demands of the brain.
3. **Extracellular Matrix:** The extracellular matrix, composed of elastin and collagen fibers, provides structural support and resilience to the arterial walls. Changes in the composition of the extracellular matrix are associated with the development of atherosclerotic plaques in carotid artery disease.

Understanding the complex interplay between the structural components and functional aspects of the carotid arteries is fundamental for unraveling the mechanisms leading to carotid artery disease. Any disturbance in the delicate balance of these elements can result in pathological changes that compromise blood flow to the brain, underscoring the clinical significance of this intricate vascular system.

Blood Supply to the Brain

The intricate network of blood vessels that supply the brain is a marvel of physiological engineering, ensuring the delivery of oxygen and nutrients essential for the organ's metabolic demands. Among these vessels, the carotid arteries play a pivotal role in maintaining cerebral perfusion, highlighting the significance of understanding the complex dynamics of blood supply to the brain.

Carotid Arteries and Brain Perfusion:

The carotid arteries, consisting of the common carotid, internal carotid, and external carotid arteries, are key contributors to the blood supply of the brain. The internal carotid arteries, in particular, are responsible for delivering blood to the anterior and middle cerebral arteries, crucial regions for cognitive function, motor control, and sensory perception.

1. **Common Carotid Artery:** Originating from the brachiocephalic trunk on the right and the aortic arch on the left, the common carotid artery ascends along the neck, bifurcating into the internal and external carotid arteries near the carotid sinus.
2. **Internal Carotid Artery (ICA):** The internal carotid artery ascends within the carotid sheath and enters the skull through the carotid canal. Inside the skull, it gives rise to the ophthalmic artery and then further bifurcates into the anterior and middle cerebral arteries, providing blood to the majority of the cerebral hemispheres.
3. **External Carotid Artery (ECA):** The external carotid artery supplies blood to the neck, face, and superficial regions of the head through various branches. While it does not directly contribute to the cerebral circulation,

the ECA's branches play a role in the collateral circulation of the scalp and face.

Collateral Circulation:

The circulatory system's redundancy is evident in the collateral circulation mechanisms that safeguard cerebral blood supply. Collateral vessels provide alternative routes for blood flow in case of partial or complete occlusion in the primary arteries, offering a protective mechanism against ischemic events.

1. **Circle of Willis:** A key component of collateral circulation in the brain is the Circle of Willis, an anastomotic circle of arteries at the base of the brain. It connects the anterior and posterior circulations, forming an essential safety net. The anterior circulation is mainly supplied by the internal carotid arteries, while the posterior circulation is primarily from the vertebral arteries.
2. **Vertebral Arteries:** The vertebral arteries, originating from the subclavian arteries, ascend through the cervical vertebrae and join to form the basilar artery. The basilar artery, in turn, contributes to the Circle of Willis and supplies the posterior cerebral arteries.

Regulation of Cerebral Blood Flow:

The brain maintains a remarkable ability to regulate its blood flow, ensuring a constant supply of oxygen and nutrients despite fluctuations in systemic blood pressure. Autoregulation is a vital mechanism that allows the cerebral vasculature to adjust its resistance in response to changes in perfusion pressure.

1. **Autoregulatory Range:** Cerebral autoregulation maintains a relatively constant blood flow within a certain range of systemic blood pressures, typically between 60 and 150 mmHg. Below or above this

range, the autoregulatory capacity may be compromised, leading to inadequate blood supply or increased risk of hemorrhage.
2. **Cerebral Autoregulation in Carotid Artery Disease:** In conditions such as carotid artery disease, where the blood supply to the brain may be compromised due to stenosis or plaque formation, the autoregulatory capacity becomes crucial. If the stenosis is severe and compromises blood flow, the brain's autoregulatory mechanisms may be challenged, increasing the vulnerability to ischemic events.

Pathophysiology of Blood Supply Disorders:

Understanding the pathophysiology of blood supply disorders to the brain is imperative for diagnosing and managing conditions like carotid artery disease.

1. **Atherosclerosis:** The primary cause of carotid artery disease is atherosclerosis, a process characterized by the accumulation of fatty deposits and plaque on the arterial walls. In the carotid arteries, this can lead to stenosis, reducing blood flow to the brain and increasing the risk of thromboembolic events.
2. **Emboli Formation:** Atherosclerotic plaques can become unstable, leading to the formation of emboli that may travel to smaller vessels in the brain, causing ischemic strokes. The internal carotid artery, being a direct supplier to the anterior and middle cerebral arteries, is particularly vulnerable to these embolic events.

In conclusion, the blood supply to the brain, orchestrated by the carotid arteries and intricately connected collateral circulations, is a marvel of physiological adaptation. Its regulation, both under normal circumstances and in the face of pathological challenges like carotid artery disease, exemplifies the body's sophisticated mechanisms for preserving cerebral perfusion and sustaining optimal brain function.

Microscopic Anatomy of Carotid Artery Walls

The microscopic anatomy of carotid artery walls provides a detailed understanding of the cellular and molecular components that contribute to the structure and function of these vital blood vessels. Composed of three distinct layers – intima, media, and adventitia – the carotid artery walls are a sophisticated amalgamation of cells, extracellular matrix, and various molecules that collectively ensure their strength, elasticity, and proper functioning.

Intima:

The intima, the innermost layer of the carotid artery wall, is a critical interface between the circulating blood and the arterial structure. Composed of endothelial cells and a supporting basement membrane, the intima serves essential roles in vascular homeostasis and regulation.

Endothelial Cells: These specialized cells form a continuous monolayer lining the interior surface of the artery. The endothelial cells play a multifaceted role in vascular function. They regulate the passage of substances between the blood and the arterial wall, produce vasodilators such as nitric oxide, and actively participate in the prevention of thrombosis by releasing anticoagulant factors.

Basement Membrane: Supporting the endothelial cells, the basement membrane provides structural integrity to the intima. It acts as a barrier and plays a role in modulating the interaction between endothelial cells and the surrounding extracellular matrix.

Media:

The media is the middle layer of the carotid artery wall and is primarily composed of smooth muscle cells (SMCs) embedded in an extracellular matrix rich in elastin and collagen fibers. This layer imparts strength, elasticity, and contractility to the artery.

Smooth Muscle Cells (SMCs): The predominant cellular component of the media, SMCs are arranged in layers around the arterial lumen. These cells are responsible for the dynamic regulation of the artery's diameter, a process crucial for maintaining blood pressure and ensuring adequate perfusion to downstream tissues, including the brain.

Extracellular Matrix (ECM): The extracellular matrix provides a structural framework for the media. It consists of proteins such as elastin, which confers elasticity, and collagen, which imparts tensile strength. The balance between these components is essential for the proper functioning of the arterial wall.

Adventitia:

The outermost layer of the carotid artery wall is the adventitia, a connective tissue layer that anchors the artery to surrounding structures. It contains blood vessels, nerves, and collagen fibers, contributing to the overall strength and resilience of the artery.

Collagen Fibers: Abundant in the adventitia, collagen fibers provide tensile strength to the artery. They form a supportive network that maintains the structural integrity of the arterial wall.

Vasa Vasorum: Small blood vessels within the adventitia, known as vasa vasorum, supply oxygen and nutrients to the outer layers of the artery. These vessels become especially critical in larger arteries where diffusion alone may be insufficient to meet the metabolic needs of the vessel wall.

Dynamic Interactions in Microscopic Anatomy:

The microscopic anatomy of carotid artery walls involves dynamic interactions between cellular components, extracellular matrix, and various signaling molecules.

1. **Vascular Smooth Muscle Cells (VSMCs) in Health:** Under normal physiological conditions, VSMCs in the media maintain a contractile phenotype. They respond to vasoactive substances, such as endothelin and angiotensin, by adjusting the arterial diameter to regulate blood flow and maintain blood pressure within a normal range.
2. **Endothelial Cell Function:** Endothelial cells actively participate in vascular homeostasis. They release nitric oxide, a potent vasodilator, in response to shear stress exerted by blood flow. Nitric oxide helps maintain vascular tone and prevents the adhesion of platelets and inflammatory cells to the endothelial surface.
3. **Extracellular Matrix Remodeling:** The balance between elastin and collagen in the extracellular matrix is crucial for arterial wall compliance. Disruptions in this balance, often associated with conditions like atherosclerosis, can lead to arterial stiffness and increased susceptibility to vascular diseases.

Pathological Alterations:

Understanding the microscopic anatomy of carotid artery walls is equally essential in the context of pathological alterations, particularly atherosclerosis.

1. **Atherosclerotic Plaque Formation:** Atherosclerosis is characterized by the accumulation of lipid-rich plaques within the intima. These plaques consist of cholesterol,

inflammatory cells, and cellular debris. As plaques grow, they can encroach upon the arterial lumen, compromising blood flow.
2. **Smooth Muscle Cell Phenotypic Switch:** In response to atherosclerotic stimuli, vascular smooth muscle cells undergo a phenotypic switch from a contractile to a synthetic state. This switch contributes to the formation of fibrous caps over atherosclerotic plaques.
3. **Endothelial Dysfunction:** Atherosclerosis is associated with endothelial dysfunction, marked by impaired nitric oxide production and increased adhesion of inflammatory cells. Endothelial dysfunction contributes to plaque formation and increases the risk of thrombotic events.

Therapeutic Implications:

Understanding the microscopic anatomy of carotid artery walls has significant therapeutic implications, particularly in the management of diseases like carotid artery stenosis.

1. **Interventional Strategies:** Therapeutic interventions for carotid artery disease often involve procedures like carotid endarterectomy or stenting. These procedures aim to remove or bypass atherosclerotic plaques, restoring proper blood flow to the brain.
2. **Pharmacological Approaches:** Medications targeting factors such as cholesterol levels, blood pressure, and antiplatelet agents play a crucial role in preventing or managing carotid artery disease. These pharmacological interventions aim to address risk factors associated with atherosclerosis and maintain vascular health.
3. **Advancements in Targeted Therapies:** Ongoing research is exploring targeted therapies that address specific molecular pathways involved in atherosclerosis. This includes medications that modulate inflammation,

stabilize atherosclerotic plaques, or promote the regression of established disease.

In conclusion, the microscopic anatomy of carotid artery walls is a complex interplay of cellular and molecular components, forming the basis for the arteries' structural integrity and physiological function. Understanding these intricate details not only enhances our knowledge of normal vascular biology but also provides critical insights into the pathological processes that underlie conditions like carotid artery disease. Such knowledge is fundamental for the development of effective therapeutic strategies aimed at preserving and restoring the health of these essential blood vessels.

Hemodynamics of Carotid Arteries

The hemodynamics of the carotid arteries refers to the study of blood flow dynamics within these crucial vessels, encompassing the principles of fluid mechanics, vessel wall interactions, and the complex interplay of forces that govern the circulatory system. Understanding the hemodynamics of the carotid arteries is fundamental to comprehending the pathophysiology of conditions such as carotid artery disease, optimizing diagnostic techniques, and developing effective therapeutic interventions.

Blood Flow Characteristics:

Blood flow within the carotid arteries is a dynamic process influenced by various factors, including vessel anatomy, cardiac output, and systemic blood pressure. The following key characteristics define the hemodynamics of blood flow in these arteries:

1. **Pulsatile Flow:** The rhythmic contraction and relaxation

of the heart result in pulsatile blood flow. During systole, blood is ejected into the arteries, causing a surge in pressure and flow. Diastole, the relaxation phase of the cardiac cycle, is characterized by decreased pressure and reduced flow.
2. **Laminar Flow:** Under normal conditions, blood flows in a laminar, streamlined fashion within the carotid arteries. This means that blood layers move parallel to each other, with faster-flowing central layers surrounded by slower peripheral layers.
3. **Reynolds Number:** The Reynolds number is a dimensionless parameter that characterizes the flow pattern of blood. In the carotid arteries, the Reynolds number is typically low, indicating that blood flow is predominantly laminar. However, certain conditions, such as stenosis or turbulence, can alter the Reynolds number and transition the flow to turbulent.

Hemodynamic Forces:

Blood flow within the carotid arteries is subject to various forces that influence its velocity, pressure, and overall dynamics. The primary hemodynamic forces include:

1. **Shear Stress:** Shear stress is the frictional force exerted by blood as it flows along the endothelial surface of the arterial wall. It plays a crucial role in maintaining vascular health by influencing endothelial function, promoting the release of vasodilators like nitric oxide, and preventing thrombosis.
2. **Pressure Gradient:** The pressure gradient, created by the difference in pressure between the proximal and distal ends of the carotid arteries, drives blood flow. This gradient ensures the continuous circulation of blood from the heart to the brain and other organs.
3. **Wall Tension:** Wall tension refers to the force exerted by

the blood on the arterial walls. It is directly proportional to blood pressure and vessel radius, highlighting the importance of maintaining optimal blood pressure to prevent excessive tension on the arterial walls.
4. **Turbulence:** While laminar flow is the norm, certain conditions, such as atherosclerosis or stenosis, can disrupt the smooth flow of blood, leading to turbulence. Turbulent flow generates additional forces and shear stress on the arterial walls, potentially contributing to vascular damage.

Effect of Vessel Geometry:

The geometric characteristics of the carotid arteries significantly impact their hemodynamics. Factors such as vessel diameter, length, and branching patterns influence blood flow dynamics in the following ways:

1. **Carotid Bifurcation:** The bifurcation of the common carotid artery into the internal and external carotid arteries is a critical site for hemodynamic considerations. The geometry of this bifurcation can influence the distribution of blood flow and the development of atherosclerotic plaques.
2. **Carotid Bulb:** The dilation or bulbous region at the carotid bifurcation is prone to disturbed flow patterns and atherosclerotic plaque formation. The complex hemodynamics in this area contribute to the vulnerability of the carotid bulb to atherosclerosis.

Impact of Atherosclerosis on Hemodynamics:

Atherosclerosis, characterized by the accumulation of plaques within the arterial walls, significantly alters the hemodynamics of the carotid arteries. The presence of atherosclerotic plaques introduces several hemodynamic changes:

1. **Stenosis and Flow Disturbances:** Atherosclerotic plaques can lead to the narrowing (stenosis) of the arterial lumen, impeding blood flow. Additionally, irregularities on the plaque surface can disrupt laminar flow, promoting turbulence and altering shear stress patterns.
2. **Increased Shear Stress at Plaque Surface:** The presence of atherosclerotic plaques can increase shear stress at the plaque surface, potentially influencing plaque stability and rupture. High shear stress may contribute to the vulnerability of certain plaques, leading to thromboembolic events.
3. **Turbulent Flow and Plaque Formation:** Turbulence generated by irregularities in the arterial wall or by the presence of atherosclerotic plaques can contribute to further plaque formation. Turbulent flow may enhance endothelial dysfunction and inflammatory responses, exacerbating the progression of atherosclerosis.

Diagnostic Techniques and Hemodynamics:

Various diagnostic techniques are employed to assess the hemodynamics of the carotid arteries, providing valuable insights into their structure and function. Key diagnostic modalities include:

1. **Doppler Ultrasound:** Doppler ultrasound is a non-invasive technique that measures blood flow velocity and direction. It is widely used to assess carotid artery hemodynamics, identify stenosis, and evaluate the presence of turbulent flow or emboli.
2. **Color Flow Imaging:** This imaging technique, often used in conjunction with Doppler ultrasound, visualizes blood flow in color-coded images. It enhances the ability to detect abnormalities such as turbulent flow or plaque formation.

3. **Magnetic Resonance Angiography (MRA):** MRA provides detailed images of the carotid arteries and surrounding structures. It can reveal the presence of atherosclerotic plaques, assess vessel geometry, and provide insights into blood flow patterns.
4. **Computed Tomography Angiography (CTA):** CTA uses X-ray technology and computer processing to generate detailed images of the carotid arteries. It is valuable for visualizing arterial anatomy, detecting stenosis, and assessing the extent of atherosclerosis.

Therapeutic Implications:

A comprehensive understanding of the hemodynamics of carotid arteries has significant therapeutic implications, particularly in the management of carotid artery disease:

1. **Surgical Interventions:** In cases of significant carotid artery stenosis, surgical interventions such as carotid endarterectomy or carotid artery stenting aim to restore proper blood flow. These procedures are guided by an understanding of the hemodynamics at play, ensuring optimal outcomes.
2. **Pharmacological Approaches:** Medications targeting factors such as blood pressure, cholesterol levels, and anticoagulation play a crucial role in influencing carotid artery hemodynamics. They are essential components of therapeutic strategies aimed at preventing progression or recurrence of carotid artery disease.
3. **Lifestyle Modifications:** Lifestyle interventions, including smoking cessation, dietary changes, and regular exercise, can positively impact carotid artery hemodynamics. These measures contribute to the overall management of cardiovascular risk factors and promote vascular health.
4. **Monitoring and Surveillance:** Regular monitoring of

carotid artery hemodynamics is essential, especially in individuals with risk factors for atherosclerosis. This enables early detection of abnormalities, allowing for timely interventions and preventive measures.

In conclusion, the hemodynamics of the carotid arteries is a dynamic and multifaceted aspect of vascular physiology. It encompasses the intricate interplay of forces, pressures, and flow patterns that are crucial for maintaining optimal blood supply to the brain. Understanding these hemodynamic principles is essential for diagnosing and managing conditions such as carotid artery disease, ensuring effective therapeutic interventions, and ultimately preserving the health and functionality of these vital blood vessels.

CHAPTER 3: ATHEROSCLEROSIS AND CAROTID ARTERY STENOSIS

Atherosclerosis Pathophysiology

Atherosclerosis is a chronic and progressive arterial disease characterized by the accumulation of lipid-rich plaques within the walls of large and medium-sized arteries. This pathological process plays a central role in the development of various cardiovascular diseases, including coronary artery disease, carotid artery disease, and peripheral arterial disease. Understanding the intricate pathophysiology of atherosclerosis is crucial for developing targeted interventions to prevent and manage this common vascular condition.

Initiation and Early Events:

The initiation of atherosclerosis involves a series of complex events that begin with damage to the endothelial cells lining the inner surface of the arteries. Endothelial dysfunction is often triggered by various risk factors, including hypertension, smoking, diabetes, and inflammation.

1. **Endothelial Dysfunction:** The healthy endothelium acts as a protective barrier, regulating vascular tone and preventing the adhesion of platelets and inflammatory cells. Endothelial dysfunction, however, compromises these functions. It leads to increased permeability, leukocyte adhesion, and a proinflammatory state, setting the stage for atherosclerosis.
2. **Low-Density Lipoprotein (LDL) Infiltration:** In response to endothelial injury, low-density lipoprotein (LDL) cholesterol particles infiltrate the subendothelial space. LDL undergoes modifications, particularly oxidation, making it more prone to uptake by macrophages.
3. **Macrophage Recruitment and Foam Cell Formation:** Macrophages attracted to the site of endothelial injury engulf the oxidized LDL particles, transforming into lipid-laden foam cells. Foam cells accumulate within the arterial wall, initiating the formation of fatty streaks – an early hallmark of atherosclerosis.

Middle Stages:

The progression of atherosclerosis involves the transformation of fatty streaks into more advanced lesions. Inflammatory processes intensify, contributing to the development of complex atherosclerotic plaques.

1. **Smooth Muscle Cell Proliferation:** As the atherosclerotic lesions progress, smooth muscle cells from the arterial media migrate into the intima. These cells proliferate and produce extracellular matrix components, contributing to the formation of a fibrous cap over the lipid-rich core.
2. **Plaque Maturation and Lipid Accumulation:** The atherosclerotic plaque continues to evolve, with ongoing accumulation of lipids, inflammatory cells, and cellular debris. The lipid core becomes more prominent, surrounded by a fibrous cap composed of smooth muscle

cells, collagen, and elastin.
3. **Plaque Vulnerability:** Plaque stability is a critical factor in atherosclerosis. Vulnerable plaques are characterized by a thin fibrous cap, a large lipid core, and increased inflammation. These plaques are prone to rupture, leading to thrombus formation and potential occlusion of the artery.

Advanced Stages:

The advanced stages of atherosclerosis involve complications such as plaque rupture, thrombosis, and the narrowing of the arterial lumen, leading to clinical manifestations.

1. **Plaque Rupture:** Vulnerable plaques are susceptible to rupture, exposing the thrombogenic lipid core to the bloodstream. This triggers the formation of a blood clot or thrombus at the site of rupture.
2. **Thrombosis and Occlusion:** The thrombus, composed of platelets, fibrin, and cellular elements, can grow and obstruct the arterial lumen. Complete occlusion of the artery may result in acute ischemic events, such as myocardial infarction, stroke, or peripheral artery disease.
3. **Calcification and Stenosis:** Over time, atherosclerotic plaques may undergo calcification, contributing to the stiffening and narrowing of the arterial walls. This calcification process further reduces the flexibility of the arteries and increases the risk of complications.

Contributing Factors:

Several risk factors and conditions contribute to the development and progression of atherosclerosis, influencing its pathophysiology:

1. **Hyperlipidemia:** Elevated levels of LDL cholesterol

and decreased levels of high-density lipoprotein (HDL) cholesterol are associated with an increased risk of atherosclerosis. The imbalance in lipid metabolism contributes to the accumulation of cholesterol within the arterial walls.

2. **Hypertension:** High blood pressure exerts chronic stress on the arterial walls, promoting endothelial dysfunction and facilitating the infiltration of lipids into the subendothelial space.

3. **Diabetes Mellitus:** Individuals with diabetes are at a higher risk of atherosclerosis due to the combination of hyperglycemia, insulin resistance, and increased inflammation. These factors contribute to endothelial dysfunction and accelerated plaque formation.

4. **Smoking:** Tobacco smoke contains harmful chemicals that directly damage endothelial cells, enhance oxidative stress, and promote inflammation. Smokers have a higher likelihood of developing atherosclerosis and experiencing adverse cardiovascular events.

5. **Inflammation:** Chronic inflammation, whether due to systemic conditions like rheumatoid arthritis or localized factors such as infections, plays a crucial role in the initiation and progression of atherosclerosis. Inflammatory mediators contribute to endothelial dysfunction and plaque instability.

Diagnostic and Imaging Techniques:

Various diagnostic techniques are employed to assess the extent and characteristics of atherosclerosis, aiding in risk stratification and therapeutic decision-making.

1. **Angiography:** Contrast angiography involves injecting a contrast dye into the arteries and obtaining X-ray images. This technique visualizes the arterial lumen and identifies areas of stenosis or occlusion.

2. **Ultrasound Imaging:** Doppler ultrasound and duplex ultrasound provide real-time images of blood flow and vessel anatomy. They are commonly used to assess carotid arteries for atherosclerosis, identifying plaques, stenosis, and flow abnormalities.
3. **Computed Tomography (CT) Angiography:** CT angiography uses X-rays to create detailed cross-sectional images of the arteries. It is valuable for visualizing the extent of atherosclerosis, particularly in coronary arteries.
4. **Magnetic Resonance Imaging (MRI):** MRI provides high-resolution images without the use of ionizing radiation. It is useful for assessing plaque composition, identifying vulnerable plaques, and evaluating the overall burden of atherosclerosis.

Preventive and Therapeutic Strategies:

Understanding the pathophysiology of atherosclerosis is crucial for implementing preventive and therapeutic strategies to mitigate its impact and reduce the risk of cardiovascular events.

1. **Lifestyle Modifications:** Healthy lifestyle choices, including a balanced diet, regular exercise, smoking cessation, and weight management, play a pivotal role in preventing and managing atherosclerosis.
2. **Cholesterol-Lowering Medications:** Statins, a class of medications, are widely used to lower LDL cholesterol levels and reduce the risk of atherosclerosis-related events. Other lipid-lowering agents may be prescribed based on individual patient profiles.
3. **Antihypertensive Medications:** Controlling hypertension is essential in managing atherosclerosis. Antihypertensive medications help maintain optimal blood pressure, reducing stress on the arterial walls.
4. **Antiplatelet Therapy:** Aspirin and other antiplatelet

medications are often prescribed to inhibit platelet aggregation, reducing the risk of thrombus formation and cardiovascular events.
5. **Diabetes Management:** Tight glycemic control in individuals with diabetes is crucial to prevent accelerated atherosclerosis. Medications and lifestyle interventions are employed to manage blood sugar levels effectively.
6. **Novel Therapies:** Ongoing research explores novel therapeutic approaches targeting inflammation, plaque stabilization, and lipid metabolism to address the complexities of atherosclerosis.

In conclusion, atherosclerosis is a multifaceted vascular disease characterized by the progressive accumulation of plaques within arterial walls. The intricate pathophysiology involves a cascade of events initiated by endothelial dysfunction, leading to lipid infiltration, inflammation, and plaque formation. Understanding the underlying mechanisms enables the development of targeted interventions aimed at preventing and managing atherosclerosis, reducing the burden of cardiovascular diseases on a global scale.

Mechanisms of Atherogenesis in Carotid Arteries

Atherogenesis, the process of atherosclerotic plaque formation, is a complex and dynamic series of events that can significantly impact the carotid arteries. These arteries, crucial for cerebral blood supply, are susceptible to atherogenesis, which involves a combination of molecular, cellular, and inflammatory processes. Understanding the mechanisms underlying atherogenesis in the carotid arteries is essential for developing targeted interventions to prevent and manage carotid artery disease.

Endothelial Dysfunction and Initiation:

1. **Endothelial Injury:** The initiation of atherogenesis in the carotid arteries often begins with endothelial injury. This injury can result from various factors such as hypertension, smoking, and oxidative stress.
2. **Loss of Endothelial Integrity:** Endothelial dysfunction leads to a loss of the normal protective functions of the endothelium, including the regulation of vascular tone and the prevention of platelet adhesion. Disruption of the endothelial barrier allows for the infiltration of lipoproteins, especially low-density lipoprotein (LDL), into the arterial wall.
3. **Oxidized LDL Uptake:** Once within the arterial wall, LDL undergoes modifications, particularly oxidation, making it more prone to uptake by macrophages. Oxidized LDL becomes a key player in the early stages of atherogenesis in the carotid arteries.

Formation of Fatty Streaks and Early Lesions:

1. **Macrophage Infiltration:** Macrophages are recruited to the site of oxidized LDL accumulation. They engulf the modified lipoproteins, transforming into foam cells. This process marks the formation of fatty streaks, the earliest visible sign of atherosclerosis.
2. **Inflammatory Response:** The presence of oxidized LDL and foam cells triggers an inflammatory response in the carotid artery walls. Inflammatory mediators, such as cytokines and chemokines, contribute to the recruitment of more immune cells, exacerbating the inflammatory milieu.
3. **Smooth Muscle Cell Activation:** Smooth muscle cells within the arterial wall become activated and migrate towards the developing atherosclerotic lesions. They

proliferate and contribute to the formation of a fibrous cap over the fatty streak, adding complexity to the lesion.

Progression to Advanced Lesions:

1. **Fibrous Cap Formation:** Over time, the atherosclerotic lesion progresses to more advanced stages. Smooth muscle cells within the plaque produce extracellular matrix components, primarily collagen. This contributes to the formation of a fibrous cap over the lipid-rich core.
2. **Lipid Core Expansion:** The lipid core within the plaque continues to accumulate cholesterol, cellular debris, and inflammatory cells. The expansion of the lipid core increases the overall size and complexity of the atherosclerotic lesion.
3. **Calcification:** In some cases, atherosclerotic plaques undergo calcification, leading to the deposition of calcium salts within the lesion. Calcification contributes to the stiffening of the plaque and may increase the risk of rupture.

Vulnerable Plaque and Complications:

1. **Thin Fibrous Cap:** Atherosclerotic plaques can develop features that render them vulnerable to complications. One key characteristic is the thinning of the fibrous cap, making the plaque more prone to rupture.
2. **Inflammation and Plaque Instability:** Persistent inflammation within the plaque contributes to its instability. Inflammatory processes weaken the fibrous cap and promote the release of enzymes that can degrade the extracellular matrix.
3. **Plaque Rupture:** The rupture of a vulnerable plaque exposes its thrombogenic contents, including tissue factor and collagen, to the bloodstream. This triggers the rapid formation of a blood clot or thrombus within the

carotid artery.

Clinical Manifestations:

1. **Thrombus Formation:** The formation of a thrombus within the carotid artery can lead to partial or complete obstruction of the vessel. Depending on the location and severity, this can result in transient ischemic attacks (TIAs) or stroke.
2. **Emboli Formation:** Atherosclerotic plaques in the carotid arteries can become a source of emboli. Fragments of plaque, thrombus, or cholesterol crystals may dislodge and travel to smaller arteries within the brain, causing ischemic events.
3. **Stenosis and Reduced Blood Flow:** Advanced atherosclerosis can lead to significant stenosis, narrowing the carotid artery lumen. This reduction in blood flow may result in ischemic symptoms, affecting cognitive function or causing transient neurological deficits.

Risk Factors and Contributing Elements:

1. **Hyperlipidemia:** Elevated levels of LDL cholesterol, especially when oxidized, contribute to the initiation and progression of atherosclerosis in the carotid arteries.
2. **Hypertension:** High blood pressure places chronic stress on the arterial walls, promoting endothelial dysfunction and facilitating the infiltration of lipids.
3. **Diabetes Mellitus:** Diabetes is associated with metabolic changes that accelerate atherogenesis, including endothelial dysfunction and increased oxidative stress.
4. **Smoking:** Tobacco smoke contains harmful substances that directly damage the endothelium, exacerbating the processes leading to atherosclerosis.
5. **Genetic Predisposition:** Genetic factors play a role in

an individual's susceptibility to atherosclerosis. Familial hypercholesterolemia and other genetic conditions may contribute to an increased risk.

Diagnostic Approaches:

1. **Carotid Ultrasound:** Non-invasive imaging techniques, such as carotid ultrasound, can visualize the carotid arteries, identify plaques, and assess blood flow. Doppler ultrasound is particularly useful in evaluating the presence and severity of stenosis.
2. **Magnetic Resonance Imaging (MRI):** MRI of the carotid arteries provides detailed images, allowing for the assessment of plaque composition, vulnerability, and overall burden.
3. **Computed Tomography Angiography (CTA):** CTA provides three-dimensional images of the carotid arteries, aiding in the identification of atherosclerotic plaques and stenosis.
4. **Angiography:** Invasive angiography involves injecting contrast dye into the carotid arteries and obtaining X-ray images, providing detailed information about the arterial lumen and the presence of atherosclerosis.

Preventive and Therapeutic Strategies:

1. **Lifestyle Modifications:** Adopting a healthy lifestyle, including a balanced diet, regular exercise, smoking cessation, and weight management, is foundational in preventing the initiation and progression of atherosclerosis in the carotid arteries.
2. **Medications:** Statins and other lipid-lowering medications are commonly prescribed to manage hyperlipidemia and reduce the risk of atherosclerotic events. Antihypertensive medications and antiplatelet agents may also be recommended.

3. **Carotid Endarterectomy:** In cases of significant carotid artery stenosis, surgical interventions such as carotid endarterectomy may be performed to remove the atherosclerotic plaque and restore proper blood flow.
4. **Carotid Artery Stenting:** Minimally invasive procedures like carotid artery stenting involve the placement of a stent to open narrowed or blocked arteries, reducing the risk of stroke.
5. **Monitoring and Regular Check-ups:** Individuals at risk for carotid artery disease should undergo regular monitoring, including imaging studies and risk factor assessments, to detect and address atherosclerosis at an early stage.

Understanding the intricate mechanisms of atherogenesis in the carotid arteries allows for the development of targeted strategies aimed at preventing, diagnosing, and managing carotid artery disease. By addressing risk factors and intervening at various stages of atherosclerosis, healthcare professionals can contribute to the preservation of vascular health and reduce the risk of debilitating cardiovascular events associated with carotid artery atherogenesis.

Role of Lipids and Lipoproteins in Atherogenesis

The intricate interplay between lipids and lipoproteins plays a central role in the development and progression of atherogenesis, particularly in the context of carotid artery disease. Lipids, including cholesterol and triglycerides, are essential components of cell membranes and serve as precursors for various signaling molecules. However, when dysregulated, elevated levels of lipids and modified lipoproteins contribute to the initiation and progression of atherosclerosis in the carotid arteries.

Lipid Metabolism:

1. **Cholesterol:** Cholesterol is a vital lipid that serves as a structural component of cell membranes and is essential for the synthesis of hormones and bile acids. There are two primary sources of cholesterol: dietary intake and endogenous production in the liver.
2. **Low-Density Lipoprotein (LDL):** LDL, often referred to as "bad cholesterol," is a lipoprotein that transports cholesterol from the liver to peripheral tissues. Elevated levels of LDL are associated with an increased risk of atherosclerosis, as excess LDL can infiltrate the arterial walls and contribute to plaque formation.
3. **High-Density Lipoprotein (HDL):** HDL, or "good cholesterol," functions in reverse cholesterol transport, removing excess cholesterol from peripheral tissues and transporting it back to the liver for excretion. High levels of HDL are generally considered protective against atherosclerosis.
4. **Triglycerides:** Triglycerides are another form of lipid that circulates in the bloodstream. Elevated triglyceride levels, often associated with dietary habits and metabolic disorders, may contribute to atherosclerosis, though their role is not as clearly defined as that of cholesterol.

Initiation of Atherogenesis:

1. **LDL Infiltration:** The initiation of atherogenesis involves the infiltration of LDL cholesterol into the subendothelial space of the arterial walls. Endothelial dysfunction, often caused by risk factors such as hypertension or smoking, facilitates the passage of LDL from the bloodstream into the arterial intima.
2. **Oxidized LDL:** Once within the arterial wall, LDL can undergo oxidative modifications, turning it into

oxidized LDL. Oxidized LDL is more prone to uptake by macrophages and triggers an inflammatory response, marking the early stages of atherosclerosis.
3. **Foam Cell Formation:** Macrophages engulf oxidized LDL, transforming into foam cells. Foam cells accumulate within the arterial walls, initiating the formation of fatty streaks – the earliest visible signs of atherosclerosis.

Role in Atherosclerotic Lesion Development:

1. **Smooth Muscle Cell Activation:** Lipids, especially oxidized LDL, contribute to the activation and migration of smooth muscle cells from the arterial media into the intima. Smooth muscle cells play a crucial role in the progression of atherosclerosis by proliferating and producing extracellular matrix components.
2. **Formation of Atherosclerotic Plaque:** The combination of lipids, inflammatory cells, and cellular debris forms atherosclerotic plaques. The plaques can evolve from fatty streaks to more advanced lesions, characterized by a lipid-rich core surrounded by a fibrous cap.
3. **Plaque Vulnerability:** Lipids continue to accumulate within the plaque, influencing its stability. A high lipid content, particularly in the form of a large lipid core, contributes to plaque vulnerability. Plaques with thin fibrous caps and a large lipid core are at an increased risk of rupture.

Impact on Inflammation and Thrombosis:

1. **Inflammatory Response:** Lipids within the plaque contribute to a persistent inflammatory response. Inflammatory mediators, released by immune cells and resident cells within the arterial walls, further exacerbate the inflammatory milieu.
2. **Thrombosis:** In advanced stages of atherosclerosis,

the interaction between lipids, inflammatory cells, and components of the plaque can lead to plaque rupture. Exposure of thrombogenic material within the plaque, such as tissue factor and collagen, triggers the rapid formation of blood clots or thrombi.
3. **Emboli Formation:** Fragments of atherosclerotic plaques, including lipid-rich material, thrombus, or cholesterol crystals, may dislodge and travel as emboli to smaller arteries within the brain. This can lead to ischemic events, contributing to the clinical manifestations of carotid artery disease.

Diagnostic Implications:

1. **Lipid Profile Testing:** Assessing lipid profiles, including levels of total cholesterol, LDL cholesterol, HDL cholesterol, and triglycerides, is a fundamental aspect of cardiovascular risk assessment. Elevated LDL cholesterol levels are associated with an increased risk of atherosclerosis.
2. **Advanced Imaging Techniques:** Advanced imaging modalities, such as magnetic resonance imaging (MRI) or computed tomography angiography (CTA), can visualize atherosclerotic plaques in the carotid arteries. These techniques aid in assessing plaque composition, vulnerability, and overall burden.

Therapeutic Approaches:

1. **Statins:** Statins are a class of medications that effectively lower LDL cholesterol levels. They are widely prescribed to manage hyperlipidemia and reduce the risk of atherosclerotic events.
2. **Antiatherogenic Medications:** Medications targeting other aspects of lipid metabolism, such as PCSK9 inhibitors, may be used to further reduce LDL cholesterol

levels and inhibit atherogenesis.
3. **Lifestyle Modifications:** Lifestyle interventions, including dietary changes, regular exercise, and smoking cessation, play a crucial role in managing lipid levels and reducing the risk of atherosclerosis.
4. **Antioxidants:** Antioxidants, such as vitamin E, may have a role in reducing oxidative stress and preventing the oxidation of LDL cholesterol. However, their clinical efficacy is a subject of ongoing research.
5. **Anti-inflammatory Agents:** Some therapeutic strategies target the inflammatory component of atherosclerosis, aiming to stabilize plaques and reduce the risk of complications.

Understanding the role of lipids and lipoproteins in atherogenesis provides valuable insights into the mechanisms underlying carotid artery disease. Therapeutic strategies that target lipid metabolism and inflammation play a pivotal role in preventing and managing atherosclerosis, ultimately contributing to the preservation of vascular health and the reduction of cardiovascular events associated with carotid artery atherogenesis.

Inflammation in Carotid Artery Disease

Inflammation is a dynamic and intricate process that plays a pivotal role in the development and progression of carotid artery disease, contributing to the initiation, growth, and complication of atherosclerotic plaques within the carotid arteries. Understanding the multifaceted aspects of inflammation in the context of carotid artery disease is essential for devising targeted therapeutic strategies and enhancing our overall approach to managing this vascular condition.

Initiation of Inflammation:

1. **Endothelial Dysfunction:** The initial stages of carotid artery disease often involve endothelial dysfunction. Various risk factors, including hypertension, smoking, and diabetes, can compromise the integrity and function of the endothelial lining, setting the stage for inflammation.
2. **Leukocyte Adhesion:** In response to endothelial dysfunction, circulating leukocytes, particularly monocytes, adhere to the dysfunctional endothelium. This adhesion is mediated by cell adhesion molecules, marking the beginning of the inflammatory cascade.
3. **Chemotaxis:** Chemotactic signals released by the damaged endothelium attract leukocytes to the site of injury within the carotid arteries. This migration of immune cells amplifies the inflammatory response and contributes to the recruitment of additional inflammatory mediators.

Inflammatory Mediators:

1. **Cytokines:** Inflammatory cytokines, such as interleukin-1 (IL-1), interleukin-6 (IL-6), and tumor necrosis factor-alpha (TNF-α), are released by activated immune cells and resident cells within the arterial walls. These cytokines propagate inflammation and orchestrate various cellular responses.
2. **Chemokines:** Chemokines play a crucial role in guiding the movement of immune cells to the inflamed areas of the carotid arteries. They act as signaling molecules, directing leukocytes to specific locations within the arterial walls.
3. **Adhesion Molecules:** Cell adhesion molecules, including vascular cell adhesion molecule-1 (VCAM-1) and

intercellular adhesion molecule-1 (ICAM-1), facilitate the adhesion and migration of leukocytes across the endothelial barrier. These molecules are upregulated in response to inflammation.

Immune Cell Infiltration:

1. **Monocytes and Macrophages:** Monocytes recruited to the inflamed areas differentiate into macrophages within the carotid arterial walls. Macrophages play a central role in the uptake of oxidized LDL cholesterol, transforming into foam cells and contributing to the formation of atherosclerotic plaques.
2. **T Lymphocytes:** T lymphocytes, specifically T-helper cells, contribute to the inflammatory milieu within the carotid arteries. They release cytokines that further activate macrophages and amplify the inflammatory response, promoting atherosclerotic lesion development.

Inflammatory Response within Atherosclerotic Plaques:

1. **Matrix Metalloproteinases (MMPs):** Inflammatory cells, particularly macrophages, release MMPs. These enzymes contribute to the degradation of the extracellular matrix within atherosclerotic plaques, potentially weakening the fibrous cap and increasing plaque vulnerability.
2. **Oxidative Stress:** Inflammation within the carotid arteries is associated with increased oxidative stress. Reactive oxygen species (ROS) generated during inflammation contribute to endothelial dysfunction, lipid oxidation, and the progression of atherosclerosis.
3. **Nuclear Factor-kappa B (NF-κB) Activation:** NF-κB is a key transcription factor that regulates the expression of genes involved in inflammation. Its activation within the carotid arterial walls enhances the production of proinflammatory mediators, contributing to a sustained

inflammatory state.

Complications and Clinical Manifestations:

1. **Plaque Rupture:** Inflammation within atherosclerotic plaques renders them vulnerable to rupture. A rupture exposes thrombogenic material to the bloodstream, initiating the formation of blood clots or thrombi within the carotid arteries.
2. **Thrombosis and Embolization:** Thrombus formation within the carotid arteries can lead to partial or complete occlusion. Fragments of thrombus or atherosclerotic plaque may break off as emboli, causing downstream ischemic events in the brain.
3. **Stenosis and Reduced Blood Flow:** Inflammatory processes contribute to the progression of atherosclerosis, leading to stenosis and the narrowing of the carotid artery lumen. Reduced blood flow may result in transient ischemic attacks (TIAs) or stroke.

Diagnostic Implications:

1. **High-Sensitivity C-Reactive Protein (hs-CRP):** Elevated levels of hs-CRP, a marker of systemic inflammation, are associated with an increased risk of cardiovascular events. Measuring hs-CRP can provide insights into the inflammatory status of individuals at risk for carotid artery disease.
2. **Imaging Modalities:** Advanced imaging techniques, such as positron emission tomography (PET) scans, can visualize areas of inflammation within the carotid arteries. Imaging inflammatory activity aids in risk stratification and may guide therapeutic decisions.

Therapeutic Strategies:

1. **Statins:** Statins, in addition to their lipid-lowering

effects, have anti-inflammatory properties. They reduce inflammation within the arterial walls and contribute to plaque stabilization.
2. **Anti-Inflammatory Medications:** Ongoing research explores the potential of anti-inflammatory medications, such as colchicine and specific monoclonal antibodies, in reducing inflammation and preventing cardiovascular events.
3. **Lifestyle Interventions:** Lifestyle modifications, including a healthy diet, regular exercise, and smoking cessation, can mitigate inflammation and contribute to the overall management of carotid artery disease.
4. **Antioxidants:** Antioxidants, such as vitamin E, may have a role in reducing oxidative stress and inflammation. However, their clinical efficacy in preventing cardiovascular events is a subject of ongoing investigation.
5. **Immunomodulatory Therapies:** Novel therapies targeting specific immune responses, including T-cell activation and cytokine production, are being explored for their potential role in modulating inflammation and atherogenesis.

Understanding the intricate role of inflammation in carotid artery disease is crucial for developing comprehensive strategies to manage this vascular condition. By targeting inflammatory processes, healthcare professionals can work towards preventing the initiation and progression of atherosclerosis, ultimately reducing the risk of complications and improving the overall outcome for individuals with carotid artery disease.

Genetic Factors in Carotid Artery Disease

Carotid artery disease, a manifestation of atherosclerosis

affecting the carotid arteries supplying blood to the brain, is influenced by a complex interplay of genetic and environmental factors. Genetic factors contribute significantly to an individual's susceptibility to atherosclerosis, impacting various aspects of lipid metabolism, inflammation, and vascular homeostasis. Understanding the genetic underpinnings of carotid artery disease is crucial for risk assessment, early detection, and the development of personalized therapeutic interventions.

Genetic Predisposition:

1. **Familial Hypercholesterolemia (FH):** FH is a hereditary disorder characterized by elevated levels of low-density lipoprotein (LDL) cholesterol. Individuals with FH have a higher risk of developing atherosclerosis, including carotid artery disease, at an earlier age.
2. **Genetic Variants in Lipid Metabolism Genes:** Specific genetic variants in genes involved in lipid metabolism, such as PCSK9, APOB, and LDLR, can influence cholesterol levels and impact the development of atherosclerosis. Understanding these variants provides insights into an individual's lipid profile and cardiovascular risk.
3. **Polymorphisms in Inflammatory Genes:** Genetic variations in inflammatory genes, including those encoding interleukins (e.g., IL-6, IL-1β) and tumor necrosis factor-alpha (TNF-α), may contribute to the modulation of the inflammatory response within the carotid arteries, influencing atherosclerotic plaque formation.
4. **Endothelial Function Genes:** Polymorphisms in genes related to endothelial function, such as eNOS (endothelial nitric oxide synthase), can affect vascular tone and responsiveness. Altered endothelial function is a key factor in the initiation of atherosclerosis.

Genetic Influence on Atherogenesis:

1. **Genes Regulating Lipid Levels:** Genetic factors play a role in determining an individual's baseline lipid profile, influencing the concentrations of LDL cholesterol, high-density lipoprotein (HDL) cholesterol, and triglycerides. Dysregulation of lipid metabolism is a key driver of atherosclerosis in the carotid arteries.
2. **Inflammatory Gene Variants:** Certain genetic variants can amplify or dampen the inflammatory response. Individuals with pro-inflammatory genetic profiles may experience heightened inflammation within the carotid arteries, potentially accelerating atherogenesis.
3. **Genetic Determinants of Plaque Stability:** The stability of atherosclerotic plaques is influenced by genetic factors. Variations in genes associated with extracellular matrix components and plaque remodeling may impact the vulnerability of plaques to rupture.
4. **Vascular Smooth Muscle Cell Function Genes:** Genetic variations affecting the function of vascular smooth muscle cells can influence their response to stimuli within the arterial walls. Changes in smooth muscle cell behavior contribute to plaque development and progression.

Gene-Environment Interactions:

1. **Gene-Diet Interactions:** The impact of genetic factors on atherosclerosis may be modulated by dietary habits. For example, individuals with specific genetic variants related to lipid metabolism may be more responsive to dietary interventions aimed at lowering cholesterol levels.
2. **Gene-Smoking Interactions:** Genetic factors can interact with environmental risk factors, such as smoking.

Smokers with certain genetic predispositions may have an increased susceptibility to endothelial dysfunction and accelerated atherosclerosis.
3. **Gene-Environment Interaction in Inflammation:** Genetic variants in inflammatory genes may interact with environmental factors, such as chronic infections or exposure to pollutants, influencing the inflammatory milieu within the carotid arteries.

Clinical Implications:

1. **Genetic Testing:** Identifying specific genetic variants associated with atherosclerosis risk can help in risk stratification. Genetic testing may reveal predispositions related to lipid metabolism, inflammation, and vascular function.
2. **Early Detection and Prevention:** Individuals with a family history of premature cardiovascular disease or known genetic risk factors may benefit from early detection strategies. Early intervention, including lifestyle modifications and targeted medications, can mitigate the impact of genetic predispositions.
3. **Personalized Treatment Approaches:** Knowledge of an individual's genetic profile allows for personalized treatment strategies. For example, individuals with familial hypercholesterolemia may require more aggressive lipid-lowering therapies.
4. **Genetic Counseling:** Individuals identified with significant genetic risks for carotid artery disease may benefit from genetic counseling. This process involves discussing the genetic basis of the condition, its inheritance patterns, and available preventive measures.
5. **Research into Novel Therapies:** Understanding the genetic factors underlying carotid artery disease is essential for ongoing research into novel therapeutic

approaches. Targeting specific genetic pathways may offer new avenues for preventing and managing the disease.

Ethical Considerations:

1. **Privacy and Informed Consent:** Genetic testing raises privacy concerns, and individuals undergoing testing should be fully informed about the implications of genetic information. Informed consent processes should address potential psychological and social implications.
2. **Equity in Access to Genetic Testing:** Ensuring equitable access to genetic testing and subsequent interventions is crucial. Disparities in access based on socioeconomic factors should be addressed to promote fair and just healthcare practices.

In conclusion, genetic factors significantly contribute to the complexity of carotid artery disease. Unraveling the genetic underpinnings of atherosclerosis enhances our understanding of disease mechanisms, facilitates risk assessment, and guides the development of personalized therapeutic approaches. The integration of genetic information into clinical practice holds promise for advancing precision medicine in the prevention and management of carotid artery disease.

CHAPTER 4: DIAGNOSIS AND IMAGING TECHNIQUES

Non-Invasive Imaging Modalities in Carotid Artery Disease

Carotid artery disease, characterized by the narrowing or blockage of the carotid arteries, poses a significant risk of stroke and other cerebrovascular events. Non-invasive imaging modalities play a crucial role in the diagnosis, risk stratification, and monitoring of carotid artery disease. This section explores three key non-invasive imaging techniques: Ultrasound (Doppler and Duplex), Magnetic Resonance Angiography (MRA), and Computed Tomography Angiography (CTA).

Ultrasound (Doppler and Duplex)

Doppler Ultrasound

Doppler ultrasound is a widely used non-invasive imaging technique that utilizes sound waves to assess blood flow within the carotid arteries. It provides valuable information about the velocity and direction of blood flow, aiding in the identification of stenosis, plaque formation, and overall vascular health.

Principle of Doppler Ultrasound:

Doppler ultrasound is based on the principle of the Doppler effect, where the frequency of sound waves changes when they encounter moving objects. In the context of carotid artery imaging, the ultrasound transducer emits sound waves that bounce off red blood cells in the bloodstream. The reflected waves are then analyzed to determine the speed and direction of blood flow.

Applications and Advantages:

1. **Stenosis Assessment:** Doppler ultrasound is particularly effective in evaluating the degree of stenosis within the carotid arteries. It can identify areas of turbulence or increased blood velocity, indicating narrowing due to atherosclerotic plaque.
2. **Plaque Characterization:** The technique allows for the visualization and characterization of atherosclerotic plaques. Plaque morphology, including size, echogenicity, and ulceration, can be assessed, contributing to risk stratification.
3. **Monitoring Blood Flow Dynamics:** Doppler ultrasound enables the real-time assessment of blood flow dynamics. Changes in velocity or the presence of turbulent flow may indicate hemodynamic alterations associated with carotid artery disease.
4. **Non-Invasiveness:** One of the significant advantages of Doppler ultrasound is its non-invasiveness. It does not involve the use of ionizing radiation or contrast agents, making it a safe and widely applicable imaging modality.
5. **Cost-Effectiveness:** Doppler ultrasound is relatively cost-effective compared to other imaging modalities, making it a practical choice for routine screening and

follow-up assessments.

Limitations and Considerations:

1. **Operator Dependence:** Doppler ultrasound is operator-dependent, and the quality of the examination may vary based on the skill and experience of the operator. Standardization and training are essential to ensure accurate and reproducible results.
2. **Limited Visualization of Vessel Wall:** While Doppler ultrasound excels in assessing blood flow, it has limitations in visualizing the vessel wall and accurately characterizing plaque composition. Additional imaging modalities may be necessary for a comprehensive evaluation.

Duplex Ultrasound

Duplex ultrasound combines traditional B-mode (brightness mode) imaging with Doppler ultrasound, providing a comprehensive assessment of both anatomical and hemodynamic aspects of the carotid arteries. This integration enhances the diagnostic capabilities of ultrasound in carotid artery disease.

Advantages and Applications of Duplex Ultrasound:

1. **Anatomical Visualization:** B-mode imaging in duplex ultrasound provides detailed anatomical images of the carotid arteries. It allows for the assessment of vessel wall thickness, the presence of plaques, and the overall structure of the arterial wall.
2. **Simultaneous Blood Flow Assessment:** By incorporating Doppler ultrasound, duplex imaging enables the simultaneous assessment of blood flow characteristics. This dual-modality approach enhances the diagnostic accuracy in detecting and characterizing carotid artery

disease.
3. **Real-Time Imaging:** Duplex ultrasound provides real-time imaging, allowing clinicians to observe blood flow patterns and plaque characteristics dynamically. This feature is particularly valuable for identifying changes during maneuvers like carotid artery compression.
4. **Risk Stratification:** The combination of anatomical and hemodynamic information allows for better risk stratification. Clinicians can assess the severity of stenosis, identify high-risk plaques, and tailor management strategies accordingly.
5. **Patient-Friendly:** Similar to Doppler ultrasound, duplex ultrasound is non-invasive and well-tolerated by patients. It does not expose individuals to ionizing radiation or contrast agents, minimizing potential risks.

Clinical Applications and Interpretation:

1. **Stenosis Grading:** Duplex ultrasound is employed for grading the severity of carotid artery stenosis. The peak systolic velocity (PSV) and end-diastolic velocity (EDV) measurements are key parameters used for this purpose. Higher velocities indicate increased blood flow resistance and potential stenosis.
2. **Plaque Morphology:** B-mode imaging in duplex ultrasound allows for the characterization of plaque morphology. Features such as echogenicity, surface irregularities, and ulcerations provide insights into plaque stability and the risk of embolization.
3. **Hemodynamic Assessment:** The spectral Doppler waveform obtained during duplex ultrasound helps assess hemodynamic changes associated with carotid artery disease. Abnormalities in waveform patterns may indicate increased turbulence or compromised blood flow.

4. **Monitoring Disease Progression:** Duplex ultrasound is valuable for monitoring disease progression over time. Serial examinations enable clinicians to track changes in stenosis severity, plaque characteristics, and blood flow dynamics.

Integration with Other Imaging Modalities:

While duplex ultrasound provides valuable information, its integration with other imaging modalities may be necessary for a comprehensive assessment. Combining ultrasound findings with those from magnetic resonance angiography (MRA) or computed tomography angiography (CTA) can offer a more detailed understanding of plaque composition and vessel wall characteristics.

Magnetic Resonance Angiography (MRA)

Magnetic Resonance Angiography (MRA) is a non-invasive imaging technique that utilizes magnetic resonance imaging (MRI) to visualize the blood vessels, including the carotid arteries. MRA provides high-resolution images without the use of ionizing radiation and is well-suited for assessing the anatomy, stenosis, and plaque composition in carotid artery disease.

Principle of MRA:

MRA relies on the principles of nuclear magnetic resonance. When the body is placed in a strong magnetic field and exposed to radiofrequency pulses, hydrogen nuclei within the body's tissues emit signals that can be detected by the MRI scanner. By manipulating these signals, MRA creates detailed images of blood vessels.

Types of MRA Techniques:

1. **Time-of-Flight (TOF) MRA:** This technique relies on

the flow-related enhancement of blood signals. It uses selective radiofrequency pulses to saturate stationary tissue signals, emphasizing blood flow signals in the vessels. TOF MRA is commonly employed for carotid artery imaging.
2. **Contrast-Enhanced MRA (CE-MRA):** Contrast agents, typically gadolinium-based, are administered intravenously to enhance the visualization of blood vessels. CE-MRA provides detailed images of the carotid arteries, highlighting areas of stenosis, plaque, and vascular anatomy.

Advantages and Applications of MRA:

1. **Detailed Anatomical Visualization:** MRA provides high-resolution, three-dimensional images of the carotid arteries, allowing for detailed visualization of the vessel lumen, plaque morphology, and the surrounding anatomy.
2. **Multi-Planar Imaging:** MRA enables imaging in multiple planes, providing a comprehensive view of the carotid arteries from various perspectives. This versatility aids in identifying complex anatomical features and accurately assessing stenosis severity.
3. **Soft Tissue Differentiation:** Magnetic resonance imaging excels in soft tissue differentiation, allowing for the characterization of plaque composition and detection of lipid-rich or hemorrhagic components within atherosclerotic plaques.
4. **No Ionizing Radiation:** Unlike computed tomography angiography (CTA), MRA does not involve ionizing radiation. This makes it a preferred choice, especially in individuals who may be more sensitive to radiation or require repeated imaging.
5. **Evaluation of Plaque Vulnerability:** MRA can contribute

to assessing plaque vulnerability by identifying features associated with high-risk plaques, such as intraplaque hemorrhage or a large lipid core.

Challenges and Considerations:

1. **Contrast-Enhanced Imaging Risks:** While gadolinium-based contrast agents used in CE-MRA are generally considered safe, there have been concerns about their potential association with nephrogenic systemic fibrosis (NSF) in individuals with impaired kidney function. Screening for renal function is typically performed before contrast administration.
2. **Availability and Cost:** MRA may be less readily available than other imaging modalities, and its cost may be higher. However, advancements in technology and increased accessibility are addressing these limitations.

Clinical Applications and Interpretation:

1. **Stenosis Grading:** MRA is effective in grading the severity of carotid artery stenosis. By visualizing the narrowing of the vessel lumen, clinicians can categorize stenosis into mild, moderate, or severe, guiding treatment decisions.
2. **Plaque Morphology:** MRA provides detailed information about plaque morphology. The identification of features such as ulcerations, calcifications, and lipid-rich components contributes to risk stratification and decision-making regarding interventions.
3. **Evaluation of Collateral Circulation:** MRA can assess collateral circulation, which may develop in response to carotid artery stenosis. Understanding collateral pathways is important for predicting the impact of stenosis on cerebral blood flow.
4. **Dynamic Contrast-Enhanced MRA:** This advanced

MRA technique involves acquiring images during the dynamic passage of a contrast agent. It provides real-time information about blood flow patterns, aiding in the assessment of vascular dynamics and potential hemodynamic significance of stenosis.
5. **Integration with Other Imaging Modalities:** MRA findings can be integrated with those from duplex ultrasound or other imaging modalities to enhance the overall understanding of carotid artery disease. Combining anatomical information from MRA with hemodynamic data from ultrasound contributes to a comprehensive assessment.

Computed Tomography Angiography (CTA)

Computed Tomography Angiography (CTA) is a non-invasive imaging modality that uses X-ray technology and computer processing to create detailed images of the blood vessels, including the carotid arteries. CTA is valuable for assessing vascular anatomy, detecting stenosis, and characterizing atherosclerotic plaques.

Principle of CTA:

CTA involves the acquisition of multiple X-ray images from different angles around the body. These images are then reconstructed using computer algorithms to create cross-sectional, three-dimensional images of the carotid arteries and surrounding structures.

Advantages and Applications of CTA:

1. **High Spatial Resolution:** CTA provides high spatial resolution, allowing for detailed visualization of the carotid arteries and accurate assessment of stenosis severity. The ability to visualize fine details makes CTA a valuable tool for anatomical assessments.

2. **Rapid Imaging:** CTA is a relatively fast imaging modality, producing images quickly. This rapid acquisition is advantageous for minimizing motion artifacts and enhancing patient comfort.
3. **Evaluation of Plaque Composition:** CTA can provide information about plaque composition, including the presence of calcifications, lipid-rich areas, and ulcerations. This information contributes to risk stratification and treatment planning.
4. **Simultaneous Assessment of Surrounding Structures:** In addition to evaluating the carotid arteries, CTA allows for the simultaneous assessment of surrounding structures, such as the skull base and neck soft tissues. This broader anatomical context is valuable for comprehensive diagnostics.
5. **Versatility in Vascular Imaging:** CTA is not limited to carotid artery imaging alone. It can be used to assess other vascular territories, providing a comprehensive overview of the arterial system in a single examination.

Challenges and Considerations:

1. **Ionizing Radiation Exposure:** One of the main considerations with CTA is the exposure to ionizing radiation. While modern CT scanners employ dose-reduction techniques, the cumulative radiation exposure should be carefully considered, especially in individuals requiring repeated imaging.
2. **Contrast Agent Use:** CTA involves the administration of iodinated contrast agents, which may pose risks for individuals with allergies, renal impairment, or other contraindications. Precautions, including hydration and screening for allergies, are taken to minimize potential complications.
3. **Calcium Blooming Artifact:** Calcified plaques within the

carotid arteries can lead to artifacts known as calcium blooming, where the presence of calcium may cause overestimation of stenosis severity. Clinicians need to be aware of this potential artifact when interpreting CTA images.

Clinical Applications and Interpretation:

1. **Stenosis Grading:** CTA is utilized for grading the severity of carotid artery stenosis, with assessments ranging from mild to severe based on the degree of luminal narrowing. The accuracy of stenosis measurements is influenced by factors such as image quality and the presence of calcifications.
2. **Plaque Characterization:** CTA allows for the characterization of atherosclerotic plaques. Differentiating between calcified and non-calcified components, as well as identifying ulcerations or irregularities, contributes to risk assessment and treatment planning.
3. **Assessment of Collateral Circulation:** CTA can provide insights into collateral circulation patterns, offering information about compensatory blood flow pathways in response to carotid artery stenosis.
4. **Evaluation of Surrounding Structures:** Beyond carotid artery assessment, CTA allows clinicians to evaluate the surrounding structures, including the presence of anatomical variations, soft tissue abnormalities, and potential sources of emboli.
5. **Correlation with Clinical Symptoms:** CTA findings are correlated with clinical symptoms, contributing to the diagnostic evaluation of individuals with suspected carotid artery disease. Understanding the relationship between imaging findings and symptomatology guides appropriate management decisions.

Integration with Other Imaging Modalities:

In clinical practice, a multimodal imaging approach is often employed for a comprehensive evaluation of carotid artery disease. Integrating CTA findings with those from other modalities, such as duplex ultrasound or MRA, enhances diagnostic accuracy and provides a more complete understanding of the disease process.

Conclusion:

Non-invasive imaging modalities, including Doppler and Duplex ultrasound, Magnetic Resonance Angiography (MRA), and Computed Tomography Angiography (CTA), play pivotal roles in the diagnosis, assessment, and monitoring of carotid artery disease. Each modality offers unique advantages and considerations, and their selection depends on factors such as clinical indications, patient characteristics, and local availability.

Doppler and Duplex ultrasound excel in providing real-time information about blood flow dynamics, stenosis severity, and plaque characteristics. These modalities are valuable for routine screening, risk stratification, and monitoring disease progression. The non-invasive nature and cost-effectiveness of ultrasound make it a practical choice for various clinical scenarios.

Magnetic Resonance Angiography (MRA) leverages the strengths of magnetic resonance imaging to offer detailed anatomical and hemodynamic information. MRA is particularly useful for assessing plaque composition, visualizing collateral circulation, and providing a comprehensive view of the carotid arteries. It is a preferred choice when avoiding ionizing radiation is a priority.

Computed Tomography Angiography (CTA) utilizes X-ray

technology to provide high-resolution images, allowing for precise assessments of stenosis severity, plaque morphology, and surrounding structures. CTA's speed and versatility make it valuable for comprehensive vascular imaging, although considerations about ionizing radiation exposure and contrast agent use are essential.

The integration of these non-invasive imaging modalities into clinical practice enables healthcare professionals to make informed decisions regarding the diagnosis and management of carotid artery disease. Advancements in technology, ongoing research, and a multidisciplinary approach contribute to the continued refinement and optimization of these imaging techniques, ultimately enhancing patient care and outcomes in the realm of cerebrovascular health.

Invasive Diagnostic Procedures in Carotid Artery Disease

Carotid artery disease, characterized by the narrowing or blockage of the carotid arteries, demands accurate and precise diagnostic approaches to guide appropriate management strategies. Invasive diagnostic procedures play a crucial role in providing detailed anatomical and functional information, aiding clinicians in assessing the severity of stenosis, identifying high-risk plaques, and determining the need for therapeutic interventions. This section explores two key invasive diagnostic procedures: Angiography and Digital Subtraction Angiography (DSA).

Angiography

Principles of Angiography

Angiography, also known as conventional angiography or catheter angiography, is an invasive imaging procedure that involves the injection of contrast dye into the blood vessels to visualize their structure and blood flow. This diagnostic technique has been a cornerstone in vascular imaging and remains a gold standard for assessing carotid artery disease due to its ability to provide high-resolution, real-time images.

Procedure Steps:

1. **Catheter Insertion:** Angiography is typically performed in a specialized suite known as an angiography suite or catheterization lab. A catheter, a thin, flexible tube, is inserted into an artery, often in the groin or wrist, and threaded through the vascular system to the carotid arteries.
2. **Contrast Injection:** Once the catheter is in position, a contrast dye is injected through the catheter directly into the carotid arteries. The contrast dye enhances the visibility of the blood vessels on X-ray images, allowing for detailed visualization of the arterial anatomy.
3. **X-ray Imaging:** X-ray images are captured in real-time as the contrast dye travels through the carotid arteries. These images provide a detailed, dynamic assessment of blood flow, stenosis, and the overall vascular architecture.

Advantages and Clinical Applications:

1. **High Spatial Resolution:** Angiography offers exceptionally high spatial resolution, allowing for precise visualization of the carotid arteries and detailed assessments of stenosis severity, plaque morphology, and collateral circulation.
2. **Real-Time Imaging:** The real-time nature of angiography provides dynamic information about blood flow patterns and allows clinicians to observe changes during maneuvers, such as carotid artery compression,

to assess hemodynamic significance.
3. **Direct Therapeutic Interventions:** In addition to its diagnostic capabilities, angiography allows for direct therapeutic interventions. Procedures such as angioplasty and stent placement can be performed during the same session if significant stenosis or vascular abnormalities are identified.
4. **Comprehensive Assessment:** Angiography enables a comprehensive assessment of the carotid arteries, including the evaluation of bifurcation anatomy, identification of complex lesions, and the visualization of vessel walls.
5. **Confirmation of Non-Invasive Findings:** In cases where non-invasive imaging modalities, such as ultrasound or MRI, provide inconclusive or discordant results, angiography serves as a confirmatory and clarifying diagnostic tool.

Challenges and Considerations:

1. **Invasiveness and Risks:** Angiography is an invasive procedure that carries inherent risks, including bleeding at the catheter insertion site, allergic reactions to contrast dye, and rare complications such as arterial dissection or embolization. Careful patient selection and appropriate pre-procedural evaluation are essential to mitigate these risks.
2. **Ionizing Radiation Exposure:** Angiography involves the use of X-rays, exposing both patients and healthcare providers to ionizing radiation. Radiation doses are carefully monitored and optimized to minimize potential harm.
3. **Contrast-Induced Nephropathy (CIN):** The use of contrast dye may pose a risk of contrast-induced nephropathy, particularly in individuals with pre-

existing kidney conditions. Adequate hydration and pre-procedural screening help reduce the likelihood of this complication.
4. **Patient Discomfort:** The catheter insertion process may cause discomfort for some patients. Conscious sedation or local anesthesia is often administered to improve patient comfort during the procedure.

Clinical Applications and Interpretation:

1. **Stenosis Grading:** Angiography allows for precise grading of carotid artery stenosis, categorizing it as mild, moderate, or severe based on the degree of luminal narrowing. This information guides decisions regarding the need for interventions such as carotid endarterectomy or angioplasty with stenting.
2. **Plaque Characterization:** Detailed imaging provided by angiography facilitates the characterization of atherosclerotic plaques. Clinicians can identify features such as ulcerations, calcifications, and the overall composition of plaques, contributing to risk stratification.
3. **Dynamic Assessment:** The dynamic nature of angiography is advantageous for assessing blood flow dynamics. Abnormalities in blood flow patterns, such as turbulence or delayed filling, may indicate the presence of stenosis or other vascular abnormalities.
4. **Therapeutic Interventions:** Angiography allows for immediate therapeutic interventions if significant stenosis or vascular lesions are identified. These interventions may include angioplasty, stent placement, or other procedures aimed at restoring normal blood flow.
5. **Follow-up Assessments:** Angiography is valuable for follow-up assessments after therapeutic interventions.

Post-procedural imaging helps verify the success of interventions, assess the patency of stents, and detect any potential complications.
6. **Integration with Non-Invasive Findings:** The information obtained from angiography is often integrated with findings from non-invasive imaging modalities, such as ultrasound or MRI, to provide a comprehensive understanding of carotid artery disease and guide patient management.

Digital Subtraction Angiography (DSA)

Principles of DSA

Digital Subtraction Angiography (DSA) is an advanced form of angiography that enhances the visualization of blood vessels by subtracting non-vascular structures from the images. DSA utilizes digital technology to acquire sequential images before and after the injection of contrast dye, allowing for the isolation of the vascular anatomy and improved detection of vascular abnormalities.

Procedure Steps:

1. **Contrast Injection and Image Acquisition:** Similar to traditional angiography, a catheter is inserted into the arteries, and contrast dye is injected. However, in DSA, a rapid sequence of X-ray images is acquired before and after the injection of contrast.
2. **Digital Subtraction Technique:** The acquired pre-contrast images are digitally subtracted from the post-contrast images, resulting in a clear visualization of the contrast-filled blood vessels without superimposed structures. This technique enhances the clarity of the vascular anatomy.

Advantages and Clinical Applications:

1. **Enhanced Vascular Visualization:** DSA provides enhanced visualization of the carotid arteries by subtracting background structures, such as bones and soft tissues, from the images. This improves the clarity of the vascular anatomy and facilitates the identification of subtle abnormalities.
2. **High Temporal Resolution:** DSA offers high temporal resolution, capturing images in rapid succession. This feature is particularly advantageous for assessing dynamic blood flow changes and detecting abnormalities during specific maneuvers or interventions.
3. **Real-Time Image Processing:** The digital subtraction technique allows for real-time image processing, enabling clinicians to visualize the vascular anatomy as it fills with contrast. This real-time feedback is valuable for making immediate decisions during interventions.
4. **Selective Imaging:** DSA allows for selective imaging of specific vascular territories. By adjusting the timing of image acquisition, clinicians can focus on the carotid arteries while minimizing radiation exposure to surrounding structures.

Challenges and Considerations:

1. **Ionizing Radiation Exposure:** Similar to traditional angiography, DSA involves the use of X-rays and carries the risk of ionizing radiation exposure. Proper dose monitoring and optimization are crucial to minimize radiation-related risks.
2. **Contrast-Induced Complications:** The use of contrast dye in DSA poses similar risks as in traditional angiography, including allergic reactions and contrast-induced nephropathy. Pre-procedural screening and appropriate hydration are essential to mitigate these risks.

3. **Procedure Duration:** While DSA provides real-time imaging, the duration of the procedure may vary based on the complexity of the case and the need for additional interventions. Prolonged procedures may increase the risk of complications.

Clinical Applications and Interpretation:

1. **Stenosis Assessment:** DSA is highly effective in assessing the severity of carotid artery stenosis. The enhanced vascular visualization and real-time image processing contribute to accurate stenosis grading, guiding decisions regarding the necessity and type of interventions.
2. **Dynamic Blood Flow Assessment:** The high temporal resolution of DSA enables dynamic assessment of blood flow patterns. Clinicians can evaluate changes in blood flow during specific maneuvers, providing insights into the hemodynamic significance of stenosis.
3. **Guidance for Interventional Procedures:** DSA is frequently used to guide interventional procedures, such as angioplasty and stent placement. Real-time imaging helps ensure precise catheter navigation, accurate placement of devices, and immediate assessment of procedural success.
4. **Identification of Vascular Abnormalities:** DSA is valuable for identifying various vascular abnormalities, including aneurysms, dissections, and other pathologies that may coexist with carotid artery disease. The ability to selectively image specific vascular territories aids in the detection of complex lesions.
5. **Post-Interventional Assessments:** DSA is utilized for post-interventional assessments, allowing clinicians to confirm the successful outcome of therapeutic procedures, assess the patency of stents, and identify any

complications that may require immediate attention.
6. **Combination with Other Imaging Modalities:** DSA findings are often integrated with those from non-invasive imaging modalities and other invasive procedures, providing a comprehensive understanding of the patient's vascular status. This multimodal approach enhances diagnostic accuracy and aids in treatment planning.

Conclusion:

Invasive diagnostic procedures, including Angiography and Digital Subtraction Angiography (DSA), play a pivotal role in the comprehensive evaluation of carotid artery disease. These procedures offer unparalleled accuracy in visualizing the vascular anatomy, assessing stenosis severity, and guiding therapeutic interventions. While the invasive nature of these procedures comes with inherent risks, their diagnostic and interventional capabilities contribute significantly to the management of individuals at risk of cerebrovascular events.

Angiography, with its high spatial resolution and real-time imaging, remains a gold standard for assessing carotid artery disease. The procedure's ability to provide dynamic information about blood flow and support direct therapeutic interventions makes it a versatile tool in the clinical setting. However, careful consideration of the risks associated with invasiveness and ionizing radiation exposure is essential.

Digital Subtraction Angiography (DSA) represents an advancement in angiographic techniques, offering enhanced vascular visualization through digital subtraction. The real-time image processing capabilities of DSA, combined with high temporal resolution, make it particularly valuable for dynamic assessments and interventional guidance. While sharing similar risks with traditional angiography, DSA's selective imaging and improved clarity contribute to its clinical utility.

The choice between non-invasive and invasive diagnostic approaches in carotid artery disease depends on various factors, including the clinical context, patient characteristics, and the specific information needed for decision-making. The integration of these diagnostic modalities into a multidisciplinary approach ensures a comprehensive understanding of the disease, facilitating personalized and effective management strategies. Advances in imaging technology, ongoing research, and a commitment to minimizing procedural risks continue to shape the landscape of invasive diagnostics in the field of cerebrovascular health.

CHAPTER 5: GRADING AND CLASSIFICATION

North American Symptomatic Carotid Endarterectomy Trial (NASCET) Criteria

The North American Symptomatic Carotid Endarterectomy Trial (NASCET) is a landmark clinical trial that significantly influenced the management and treatment decisions for carotid artery disease, specifically focusing on symptomatic patients. The trial, conducted in the 1990s, aimed to assess the efficacy of carotid endarterectomy (CEA) in reducing the risk of stroke in individuals with symptomatic carotid artery stenosis. The NASCET criteria were established to standardize the assessment of carotid artery stenosis severity based on angiographic imaging findings.

Background and Objectives

The initiation of the NASCET was prompted by the need to evaluate the role of surgical intervention, specifically carotid endarterectomy, in reducing the risk of stroke in patients with symptomatic carotid artery disease. The trial included individuals who had experienced recent transient ischemic attacks (TIAs) or non-cardioembolic strokes attributable to ipsilateral carotid artery stenosis. The primary objective was to determine whether CEA was more beneficial than medical management alone in preventing future strokes.

NASCET Criteria for Stenosis Grading

The NASCET criteria established a standardized method for grading the severity of carotid artery stenosis based on angiographic imaging. The degree of stenosis was determined by measuring the narrowest diameter of the internal carotid artery (ICA) at the point of maximal stenosis and comparing it to the diameter of the normal, adjacent distal internal carotid artery.

The NASCET criteria defined four specific categories of stenosis:

1. **Normal:** No visible stenosis or minimal irregularities in the arterial lumen.
2. **Mild Stenosis:** Stenosis occupying less than 29% of the lumen diameter.
3. **Moderate Stenosis:** Stenosis ranging from 30% to 69% of the lumen diameter.
4. **Severe Stenosis or Occlusion:** Stenosis occupying 70% or more of the lumen diameter or complete occlusion.

Role in Clinical Decision-Making

The NASCET criteria have played a pivotal role in guiding clinical decision-making, especially regarding the selection of patients for carotid endarterectomy. The trial demonstrated a significant reduction in the risk of ipsilateral stroke for patients with symptomatic carotid artery stenosis exceeding 70% who underwent CEA compared to those managed medically.

The key findings of NASCET influenced the following recommendations:

1. **CEA for Severe Stenosis:** Patients with symptomatic carotid artery stenosis exceeding 70% as per NASCET criteria were identified as a group that significantly

benefited from carotid endarterectomy. The trial demonstrated a substantial absolute risk reduction in the occurrence of ipsilateral stroke for this subgroup undergoing surgical intervention.
2. **Medical Management for Mild to Moderate Stenosis:** Patients with mild to moderate stenosis (less than 70%) did not demonstrate a clear benefit from carotid endarterectomy. As a result, medical management, including antiplatelet therapy and risk factor modification, became the standard approach for this subgroup.
3. **Individualized Decision-Making:** The NASCET criteria, while providing valuable guidance, underscored the importance of individualized decision-making. Factors such as patient age, comorbidities, and life expectancy were recognized as crucial considerations in determining the most appropriate management strategy for each patient.

Limitations and Ongoing Relevance

Despite its significant impact on clinical practice, the NASCET criteria have some limitations. The criteria are primarily based on angiographic assessments, and the applicability of these findings to real-world clinical scenarios may vary. The criteria do not account for additional factors that may influence treatment decisions, such as plaque morphology, ulceration, or the presence of collateral circulation.

Moreover, advancements in imaging modalities, including non-invasive techniques such as ultrasound, magnetic resonance angiography (MRA), and computed tomography angiography (CTA), have expanded the armamentarium for assessing carotid artery disease. These modalities provide detailed information about plaque morphology, vessel wall characteristics, and overall vascular health, contributing to a more comprehensive evaluation.

Nevertheless, the NASCET criteria remain relevant in the context of their historical significance and the foundational role they played in shaping the understanding of carotid artery disease. While subsequent trials and advancements in imaging technology have refined the assessment of carotid artery stenosis, the NASCET criteria laid the groundwork for evidence-based decision-making and the establishment of treatment guidelines for patients with symptomatic carotid artery disease.

In contemporary practice, the NASCET criteria continue to inform discussions between healthcare providers and patients regarding the potential benefits and risks of carotid endarterectomy. The ongoing relevance of these criteria emphasizes the importance of a multidisciplinary approach, incorporating both historical evidence and contemporary insights, to optimize the care and outcomes of individuals with carotid artery disease.

European Carotid Surgery Trial (ECST) Criteria

The European Carotid Surgery Trial (ECST) represents another pivotal clinical trial that significantly contributed to the understanding and management of carotid artery disease. Similar to the North American Symptomatic Carotid Endarterectomy Trial (NASCET), ECST focused on evaluating the efficacy of carotid endarterectomy (CEA) in preventing strokes in patients with carotid artery stenosis. The trial provided specific criteria for grading the severity of carotid stenosis based on angiographic imaging, offering additional insights into the optimal management of this condition.

Background and Objectives

The ECST, conducted in Europe during the same era as NASCET, shared a common goal of assessing the role of carotid endarterectomy in reducing the risk of stroke in individuals with carotid artery stenosis. The trial included both symptomatic and asymptomatic patients, aiming to provide comprehensive evidence on the benefits of surgical intervention.

ECST Criteria for Stenosis Grading

Similar to NASCET, the ECST established criteria for the standardized grading of carotid artery stenosis based on angiographic imaging. The degree of stenosis was determined by measuring the narrowest diameter of the internal carotid artery (ICA) at the point of maximal stenosis and comparing it to the diameter of the normal, adjacent distal internal carotid artery.

The ECST criteria defined four specific categories of stenosis:

1. **Normal or Minimal Stenosis:** No visible stenosis or stenosis occupying less than 29% of the lumen diameter.
2. **Moderate Stenosis:** Stenosis ranging from 30% to 69% of the lumen diameter.
3. **Severe Stenosis:** Stenosis occupying 70% to 99% of the lumen diameter.
4. **Occlusion:** Complete occlusion of the internal carotid artery.

Comparison with NASCET Criteria

While the ECST criteria share similarities with NASCET in terms of stenosis grading, there are some differences in the categorization, particularly in the definition of severe stenosis. The ECST criteria include stenosis up to 99% in the severe category, whereas NASCET specifically reserves the severe category for stenosis occupying 70% or more of the lumen diameter.

These differences highlight the variations that existed in the categorization of stenosis severity during the era of these trials. It is essential for clinicians to be aware of these distinctions when interpreting and applying the findings from studies that utilized either set of criteria.

Clinical Implications and Decision-Making

The ECST criteria, much like the NASCET criteria, significantly influenced clinical decision-making regarding the management of carotid artery disease. The trial's findings, combined with those of NASCET, contributed to the establishment of evidence-based guidelines for the selection of patients for carotid endarterectomy.

Key clinical implications of the ECST criteria include:

1. **CEA for Severe Stenosis:** The ECST, similar to NASCET, supported the efficacy of carotid endarterectomy in reducing the risk of stroke for patients with severe carotid artery stenosis. Surgical intervention was found to be particularly beneficial for individuals with stenosis exceeding 70%.
2. **Medical Management for Moderate Stenosis:** Patients with moderate stenosis (30% to 69%) did not demonstrate a clear benefit from carotid endarterectomy in terms of stroke prevention. Medical management, including antiplatelet therapy and risk factor modification, was considered the standard approach for this subgroup.
3. **Individualized Decision-Making:** As emphasized by both ECST and NASCET, individualized decision-making remains crucial. Factors such as patient age, comorbidities, and overall life expectancy should be carefully considered when determining the most

appropriate management strategy for each patient.

Limitations and Ongoing Relevance

While the ECST criteria provided valuable insights into the management of carotid artery disease, similar limitations as those of NASCET exist. The criteria primarily rely on angiographic assessments and do not encompass additional factors, such as plaque composition and morphology, which may influence treatment decisions.

Advancements in imaging technology, including non-invasive modalities like ultrasound, magnetic resonance angiography (MRA), and computed tomography angiography (CTA), have expanded the array of available diagnostic tools. These modalities offer detailed information about plaque characteristics, allowing for a more comprehensive evaluation of carotid artery disease.

Despite these advancements, the ECST criteria retain historical significance and continue to contribute to the foundation of evidence guiding the management of carotid artery disease. The ongoing relevance of these criteria underscores the importance of a comprehensive, multidisciplinary approach that incorporates historical evidence and contemporary insights into the decision-making process.

In conclusion, the European Carotid Surgery Trial (ECST) criteria, along with the North American Symptomatic Carotid Endarterectomy Trial (NASCET) criteria, have played instrumental roles in shaping the understanding and management of carotid artery disease. These criteria have provided valuable guidance for clinicians in determining the optimal treatment strategies for patients with varying degrees of carotid artery stenosis, highlighting the importance of evidence-based, individualized care in the field of vascular health.

Asymptomatic Carotid Artery Stenosis

Asymptomatic carotid artery stenosis refers to the presence of narrowed or blocked carotid arteries in individuals who do not exhibit symptoms related to the condition. The carotid arteries, located on either side of the neck, supply blood to the brain. Stenosis, or narrowing of these arteries, can result from the buildup of atherosclerotic plaque, a condition known as atherosclerosis. While symptomatic carotid artery stenosis is associated with a higher risk of stroke or transient ischemic attack (TIA), asymptomatic stenosis presents a unique set of considerations in terms of diagnosis, risk stratification, and management.

Diagnosis and Assessment

Diagnosing asymptomatic carotid artery stenosis often involves imaging studies to evaluate the extent of narrowing and assess the risk of future cerebrovascular events. Common diagnostic modalities include:

1. **Duplex Ultrasound:** Duplex ultrasound is a non-invasive imaging technique that combines traditional ultrasound with Doppler ultrasound. It provides real-time images of blood flow in the carotid arteries, helping assess the degree of stenosis and identify the presence of plaque.
2. **Magnetic Resonance Angiography (MRA):** MRA utilizes magnetic resonance imaging to create detailed images of the carotid arteries. It offers information about the vessel anatomy, plaque composition, and blood flow characteristics without exposing the patient to ionizing radiation.
3. **Computed Tomography Angiography (CTA):** CTA uses X-ray technology to generate detailed images of the carotid

arteries. It provides information about stenosis severity, plaque morphology, and the surrounding vascular structures.

4. **Carotid Artery Ultrasonography:** This test involves using high-frequency sound waves to create images of the carotid arteries. It is particularly useful for assessing plaque characteristics, including size, location, and composition.

The choice of diagnostic modality depends on factors such as availability, patient characteristics, and the need for detailed information about plaque morphology.

Risk Stratification

Risk stratification is crucial in determining the appropriate management strategy for individuals with asymptomatic carotid artery stenosis. Several factors influence the risk of future cerebrovascular events:

1. **Degree of Stenosis:** The severity of stenosis, often expressed as a percentage of luminal narrowing, is a key determinant of risk. Generally, mild to moderate stenosis may pose a lower risk compared to severe stenosis.
2. **Plaque Characteristics:** The composition of atherosclerotic plaques, including features like ulceration, calcification, and lipid content, can influence the risk of plaque rupture and embolization.
3. **Age and Comorbidities:** Advanced age and the presence of other cardiovascular risk factors, such as hypertension, diabetes, and smoking, contribute to an individual's overall vascular risk.
4. **Contralateral Carotid Artery Status:** The condition of the contralateral carotid artery is considered in risk assessment. Bilateral carotid artery involvement may increase the overall risk of events.

Risk stratification aids in identifying individuals who may benefit from more aggressive interventions, such as carotid endarterectomy or carotid artery stenting, versus those for whom conservative management and medical therapy are sufficient.

Management Approaches

The management of asymptomatic carotid artery stenosis involves a multidisciplinary approach, considering both medical and interventional strategies:

1. **Medical Management:**
   - **Antiplatelet Therapy:** Aspirin or other antiplatelet medications are often prescribed to reduce the risk of clot formation in the narrowed arteries.
   - **Statins:** Statin medications may be recommended to lower cholesterol levels and stabilize plaques, potentially reducing the risk of plaque rupture.
   - **Blood Pressure Control:** Effective management of blood pressure is crucial in minimizing the risk of cardiovascular events.
2. **Lifestyle Modifications:**
   - **Smoking Cessation:** Smoking is a significant risk factor for atherosclerosis and cardiovascular events. Quitting smoking is a crucial component of preventive care.
   - **Dietary Changes:** Adopting a heart-healthy diet low in saturated fats, cholesterol, and sodium can contribute to overall cardiovascular health.
   - **Regular Exercise:** Regular physical activity supports cardiovascular health and can help manage risk factors such as hypertension and obesity.

3. **Interventional Approaches:**
   - **Carotid Endarterectomy (CEA):** In selected cases with high-grade stenosis and favorable anatomy, CEA may be considered to surgically remove the plaque and restore normal blood flow.
   - **Carotid Artery Stenting (CAS):** This minimally invasive procedure involves placing a stent in the narrowed segment of the carotid artery to improve blood flow.

Ongoing Monitoring and Follow-Up

Individuals with asymptomatic carotid artery stenosis require regular monitoring to assess the effectiveness of management strategies and detect any changes in the disease progression. Follow-up imaging studies, such as duplex ultrasound or MRA, may be performed at intervals determined by the treating healthcare provider.

Ongoing risk factor management, medication adherence, and lifestyle modifications are integral components of long-term care. The frequency and intensity of monitoring may be adjusted based on individual responses to treatment and changes in clinical status.

Shared Decision-Making

Shared decision-making between healthcare providers and individuals with asymptomatic carotid artery stenosis is essential. The potential benefits and risks of interventions, as well as the impact on quality of life, should be thoroughly discussed. Factors such as patient preferences, values, and individualized risk assessments contribute to the development of a personalized care plan.

In conclusion, the management of asymptomatic carotid artery stenosis involves a comprehensive and individualized approach that considers diagnostic findings, risk stratification, and a combination of medical and interventional strategies. Ongoing monitoring and shared decision-making are key elements in optimizing outcomes for individuals with this condition, emphasizing the importance of a patient-centered approach to vascular health.

CHAPTER 6: NATURAL HISTORY OF CAROTID ARTERY STENOSIS

Progression of Atherosclerosis

Atherosclerosis is a dynamic and complex vascular disease characterized by the accumulation of lipids, inflammatory cells, and fibrous tissue within arterial walls. Understanding the progression of atherosclerosis is crucial for developing effective preventive and therapeutic strategies. The process involves several stages, each contributing to the development and complications of atherosclerotic lesions.

Initiation of Atherosclerosis

The initiation of atherosclerosis begins with endothelial dysfunction, where the inner lining of blood vessels, the endothelium, undergoes changes that compromise its normal function. Various factors, including hypertension, smoking, hyperlipidemia, and diabetes, contribute to endothelial dysfunction.

1. **Endothelial Dysfunction:** Increased oxidative stress and inflammation impair endothelial function, reducing its ability to regulate vascular tone and permeability.

Dysfunction allows for the entry of lipids, especially low-density lipoproteins (LDL), into the arterial wall.
2. **Formation of Fatty Streaks:** LDL cholesterol undergoes modification within the arterial intima, attracting monocytes and macrophages. These cells engulf modified LDL, transforming into foam cells. The initial accumulation of foam cells results in fatty streaks, the earliest visible sign of atherosclerosis.

Progression to Intermediate Lesions

Fatty streaks can progress to more advanced lesions, known as intermediate lesions, through a series of events involving inflammation, smooth muscle cell migration, and the formation of a fibrous cap.

1. **Inflammatory Response:** Ongoing inflammation leads to the recruitment of immune cells, including T lymphocytes, contributing to the inflammatory milieu within the plaque.
2. **Smooth Muscle Cell Migration:** Smooth muscle cells within the arterial wall migrate into the developing plaque. These cells proliferate and produce extracellular matrix components, contributing to the formation of a fibrous cap.
3. **Formation of Fibrous Cap:** The fibrous cap, composed of smooth muscle cells, collagen, and elastin, overlays the lipid-rich core of the atherosclerotic plaque. This cap provides structural stability to the lesion.

Development of Advanced Atherosclerotic Lesions

Advanced atherosclerotic lesions are characterized by the progression of fibrous cap formation, the accumulation of a necrotic core, and the potential for complications such as plaque rupture or erosion.

1. **Necrotic Core Formation:** The central region of the plaque undergoes necrosis as a result of apoptosis and death of foam cells. The necrotic core is rich in lipid debris and cellular remnants.
2. **Plaque Calcification:** Calcium deposits may accumulate within the plaque, contributing to its stability but also making it more rigid and less resilient.
3. **Vulnerable Plaque:** Atherosclerotic plaques may become vulnerable to rupture or erosion, especially when the fibrous cap is thin, and inflammation is intense. Rupture exposes the thrombogenic material within the plaque to the bloodstream, leading to thrombus formation.

Complications and Clinical Consequences

Complications arising from advanced atherosclerosis can have severe clinical consequences, such as acute coronary syndromes, strokes, or peripheral artery disease.

1. **Plaque Rupture:** Rupture of a vulnerable plaque exposes the underlying thrombogenic material, triggering platelet activation and thrombus formation. The resulting thrombus may partially or completely obstruct the artery.
2. **Thrombosis and Embolization:** Thrombi formed on the surface of a ruptured plaque can cause complete occlusion of the vessel or embolize to distant sites, leading to acute cardiovascular events.
3. **Stenosis and Ischemia:** Progressive plaque growth and luminal narrowing contribute to chronic vessel stenosis, limiting blood flow to downstream tissues and organs. Ischemia may manifest as angina in coronary arteries or claudication in peripheral arteries.

Regression and Stabilization

While atherosclerosis is generally considered a progressive

disease, interventions and lifestyle modifications can promote regression or stabilization of plaques.

1. **Lifestyle Modifications:** Adopting a heart-healthy lifestyle, including a balanced diet, regular physical activity, smoking cessation, and blood pressure control, can positively impact lipid profiles and reduce cardiovascular risk.
2. **Pharmacological Interventions:** Medications such as statins, which lower cholesterol levels and possess anti-inflammatory properties, may contribute to plaque stabilization and regression.
3. **Interventional Procedures:** In some cases, procedures like percutaneous coronary intervention (PCI) or carotid endarterectomy may be performed to alleviate stenosis and reduce the risk of complications.

6 Future Directions and Research

Ongoing research explores novel therapeutic targets, imaging modalities, and personalized approaches for managing atherosclerosis. Understanding the molecular mechanisms and genetic factors influencing atherosclerosis may lead to more targeted interventions and preventive strategies.

In conclusion, the progression of atherosclerosis involves a series of complex and interrelated events, from the initiation of endothelial dysfunction to the development of advanced plaques with the potential for complications. Comprehensive strategies focusing on lifestyle modifications, pharmacological interventions, and, when necessary, interventional procedures are crucial for managing atherosclerosis and reducing the associated cardiovascular risks. Ongoing research continues to refine our understanding of the disease, offering hope for more effective and personalized approaches in the future.

Factors Influencing Disease Progression in Atherosclerosis

The progression of atherosclerosis is influenced by a multitude of factors, encompassing genetic, environmental, and lifestyle components. Understanding these factors is essential for developing targeted interventions and preventive strategies. The interplay of various elements contributes to the complexity of atherosclerotic disease progression.

Risk Factors: Traditional and Emerging

1. **Traditional Risk Factors:**
    - **Hyperlipidemia:** Elevated levels of low-density lipoprotein (LDL) cholesterol, especially when oxidized, contribute to the initiation and progression of atherosclerosis.
    - **Hypertension:** Chronic high blood pressure damages the endothelium, promoting the entry of lipids into the arterial wall and accelerating atherosclerosis.
    - **Smoking:** Tobacco smoke contains toxins that induce endothelial dysfunction, increase inflammation, and enhance the formation of atherosclerotic plaques.
    - **Diabetes Mellitus:** Diabetes accelerates atherosclerosis through mechanisms involving insulin resistance, inflammation, and oxidative stress.
2. **Emerging Risk Factors:**
    - **Inflammatory Markers:** Elevated levels of inflammatory markers, such as C-reactive protein (CRP), contribute to plaque destabilization and progression.

- **Lipoprotein(a) [Lp(a)]:** Elevated Lp(a) levels are associated with an increased risk of atherosclerotic events and may contribute to plaque formation.

Genetics and Familial Predisposition

1. **Genetic Factors:**
    - **Genetic Predisposition:** Familial hypercholesterolemia and other genetic conditions influence lipid metabolism and contribute to atherosclerosis.
    - **Polymorphisms and Gene Variants:** Variations in genes involved in lipid metabolism, inflammation, and endothelial function may influence susceptibility to atherosclerosis.

Inflammatory Pathways and Immune Responses

1. **Inflammation:**
    - **Chronic Inflammation:** Persistent inflammatory processes within the arterial wall contribute to plaque formation and progression.
    - **Immune Cell Activation:** Infiltration of immune cells, particularly macrophages and T lymphocytes, accelerates plaque development and destabilization.

Hemodynamic Factors and Shear Stress

1. **Hemodynamic Forces:**
    - **Shear Stress:** Disturbed blood flow patterns, low shear stress, and turbulent flow at arterial bifurcations contribute to endothelial dysfunction and plaque formation.
    - **Hemodynamic Stress:** High blood pressure and

hemodynamic stress on arterial walls exacerbate endothelial damage and promote atherosclerosis.

Plaque Characteristics and Composition

1. **Plaque Features:**
   - **Vulnerable Plaques:** Plaques with a thin fibrous cap, large lipid core, and increased inflammatory activity are more prone to rupture and thrombosis.
   - **Calcification:** The presence of calcified deposits can stabilize plaques but may also increase their vulnerability.

6 Lifestyle and Environmental Influences

1. **Dietary Habits:**
   - **High-Fat and High-Cholesterol Diet:** Diets rich in saturated fats and cholesterol contribute to elevated LDL cholesterol levels and atherosclerosis.
   - **Antioxidant-Rich Diets:** Consumption of fruits, vegetables, and foods with antioxidant properties may have a protective effect against oxidative stress.
2. **Physical Activity:**
   - **Regular Exercise:** Physical activity promotes cardiovascular health by improving lipid profiles, reducing inflammation, and enhancing endothelial function.
3. **Psychosocial Factors:**
   - **Stress and Mental Health:** Chronic stress and mental health conditions may contribute to atherosclerosis through mechanisms involving inflammation and lifestyle behaviors.

Aging and Hormonal Influences

1. **Aging:**
   - **Vascular Aging:** The aging process is associated with structural changes in blood vessels, making them more susceptible to atherosclerosis.
2. **Hormonal Factors:**
   - **Estrogen and Testosterone:** Hormonal fluctuations, particularly in postmenopausal women, may influence the progression of atherosclerosis.

Coagulation and Thrombosis

1. **Thrombotic Tendencies:**
   - **Prothrombotic States:** Conditions promoting hypercoagulability, such as elevated levels of clotting factors, increase the risk of thrombus formation on vulnerable plaques.

Metabolic Syndrome and Obesity

1. **Metabolic Factors:**
   - **Metabolic Syndrome:** Clusters of metabolic abnormalities, including abdominal obesity, insulin resistance, and dyslipidemia, contribute to atherosclerosis.
2. **Obesity:**
   - **Adipose Tissue Inflammation:** Inflammation associated with obesity, particularly visceral fat, exacerbates atherosclerosis.

Environmental Exposures

1. **Air Pollution:**
   - **Particulate Matter and Environmental Toxins:**

Exposure to air pollutants contributes to oxidative stress and inflammation, promoting atherosclerosis.

Medications and Therapeutic Interventions

1. **Medications:**
   - **Statins and Lipid-Lowering Drugs:** Statins reduce LDL cholesterol and possess anti-inflammatory properties, impacting the progression of atherosclerosis.
   - **Antihypertensive Medications:** Controlling blood pressure with medications helps mitigate the impact of hypertension on arterial walls.
2. **Interventions:**
   - **Percutaneous Interventions:** Procedures like angioplasty and stent placement may be performed to alleviate severe stenosis and reduce the risk of complications.

Interactions and Synergies

1. **Multifactorial Nature:**
   - **Interaction of Factors:** Atherosclerosis results from the intricate interplay of multiple factors, and their combined effects may synergistically accelerate disease progression.

Personalized Medicine and Risk Stratification

1. **Individualized Approach:**
   - **Risk Stratification:** Tailoring interventions based on individual risk profiles and genetic predispositions enables a more personalized approach to atherosclerosis management.

Understanding the complex network of factors influencing

the progression of atherosclerosis is essential for developing comprehensive strategies for prevention, early detection, and targeted interventions. A holistic approach that addresses multiple risk factors and considers individual variability is crucial for optimizing outcomes and reducing the burden of atherosclerotic cardiovascular disease. Ongoing research continues to refine our understanding of these factors and explore new avenues for therapeutic interventions.

Complications and Sequelae of Atherosclerosis

Atherosclerosis, a chronic inflammatory condition characterized by the buildup of plaque within arteries, can lead to a range of complications and sequelae, significantly impacting cardiovascular health. Understanding these consequences is crucial for developing effective management and preventive strategies. The complications of atherosclerosis encompass acute events and chronic conditions that can result from the progression of the disease.

Acute Complications

1. **Myocardial Infarction (Heart Attack):**
    - **Pathophysiology:** Rupture of a vulnerable plaque can trigger the formation of a thrombus, leading to the sudden blockage of a coronary artery. This results in the inadequate blood supply to a portion of the heart muscle, causing myocardial infarction.
    - **Clinical Manifestations:** Symptoms include chest pain or discomfort, shortness of breath, and sweating. Prompt medical intervention, such as percutaneous coronary intervention (PCI) or thrombolytic therapy, is essential to restore blood

flow and minimize myocardial damage.

2. **Stroke (Cerebrovascular Accident):**
   - **Ischemic Stroke:** Plaque rupture or embolization of a thrombus from a carotid artery plaque can result in the obstruction of cerebral blood vessels, leading to an ischemic stroke.
   - **Hemorrhagic Stroke:** Rupture of an atherosclerotic artery within the brain can cause bleeding, leading to a hemorrhagic stroke.
   - **Clinical Manifestations:** Symptoms may include sudden weakness, numbness, speech difficulties, or loss of consciousness. Timely intervention, such as thrombolytic therapy or mechanical thrombectomy, is crucial for stroke management.

3. **Acute Limb Ischemia:**
   - **Peripheral Artery Thrombosis:** Atherosclerotic plaques in peripheral arteries may rupture, leading to the formation of a thrombus and acute limb ischemia.
   - **Clinical Manifestations:** Symptoms include severe pain, pallor, coldness, and loss of pulses in the affected limb. Urgent intervention, such as thrombolysis or surgical revascularization, is necessary to restore blood flow.

Chronic Complications

1. **Coronary Artery Disease (CAD):**
   - **Chronic Ischemic Heart Disease:** Progressive narrowing of coronary arteries due to atherosclerosis can result in chronic ischemic heart disease, leading to symptoms such as angina (chest pain or discomfort) during physical exertion or emotional stress.
   - **Heart Failure:** Advanced CAD can contribute to

the development of heart failure, where the heart's pumping ability is compromised.

2. **Peripheral Artery Disease (PAD):**
   - **Claudication:** Atherosclerosis affecting the arteries supplying the lower extremities can result in intermittent claudication, characterized by pain or cramping in the legs during walking or physical activity.
   - **Critical Limb Ischemia:** Severe PAD may progress to critical limb ischemia, with persistent pain at rest, non-healing wounds, and a risk of limb loss.
3. **Aortic Aneurysm:**
   - **Abdominal Aortic Aneurysm (AAA) or Thoracic Aortic Aneurysm:** Atherosclerosis can weaken the walls of the aorta, leading to the development of an aneurysm. Rupture of an aneurysm can be life-threatening.
   - **Clinical Manifestations:** Aneurysms are often asymptomatic but can present with abdominal or back pain in the case of AAA.
4. **Chronic Renal Disease:**
   - **Renal Artery Stenosis:** Atherosclerosis affecting the renal arteries can lead to renal artery stenosis, contributing to chronic kidney disease.
   - **Clinical Manifestations:** Hypertension and declining renal function may result from reduced blood flow to the kidneys.

Systemic Complications

1. **Systemic Atherosclerosis:**
   - **Multi-Organ Involvement:** Atherosclerosis is a systemic disease that can affect arteries throughout the body, contributing to multi-organ complications.

- **Clinical Manifestations:** Systemic manifestations may include hypertension, impaired cognitive function, and impaired blood flow to various organs.

2. **Coronary Microvascular Dysfunction:**
    - **Microvascular Angina:** Atherosclerosis can also affect the smaller coronary vessels, leading to microvascular dysfunction and symptoms of angina without significant obstructive coronary artery disease.
    - **Clinical Manifestations:** Patients may experience chest pain or discomfort, often triggered by exertion or stress.

Thromboembolic Events

1. **Peripheral Embolization:**
    - **Embolization of Plaque Material:** Fragments of atherosclerotic plaques can embolize and travel to distant arteries, leading to thromboembolic events.
    - **Clinical Manifestations:** Emboli may occlude arteries in various organs, resulting in transient ischemic attacks (TIAs) or organ-specific ischemic events.

Cardiovascular Events in Diabetic Patients

1. **Diabetic Vasculopathy:**
    - **Accelerated Atherosclerosis:** Individuals with diabetes mellitus are at an increased risk of accelerated atherosclerosis and cardiovascular events.
    - **Clinical Implications:** Diabetic vasculopathy contributes to a higher incidence of coronary artery disease, stroke, and peripheral artery

disease in diabetic patients.

6 Psychological and Quality of Life Impact

1. **Psychosocial Consequences:**
   - **Quality of Life:** Chronic conditions associated with atherosclerosis, such as heart failure or chronic limb ischemia, can significantly impact an individual's quality of life.
   - **Psychological Distress:** Living with the uncertainty of cardiovascular complications may lead to psychological distress, anxiety, and depression.

Mortality and Life Expectancy

1. **Cardiovascular Mortality:**
   - **Leading Cause of Death:** Atherosclerosis-related complications, especially myocardial infarction and stroke, contribute to a significant proportion of cardiovascular mortality worldwide.
2. **Reduced Life Expectancy:**
   - **Impact on Life Expectancy:** Atherosclerosis, if left uncontrolled, can reduce life expectancy due to the increased risk of acute cardiovascular events and complications.

Understanding the diverse complications and sequelae of atherosclerosis emphasizes the importance of preventive measures, early detection, and comprehensive management strategies. Lifestyle modifications, risk factor control, and targeted interventions play crucial roles in mitigating the impact of atherosclerotic disease on cardiovascular health and overall well-being. Patient education, regular medical monitoring, and a collaborative approach between healthcare providers and individuals at risk are essential components of effective atherosclerosis management.

CHAPTER 7: MEDICAL MANAGEMENT

Lifestyle Modifications in the Management of Carotid Artery Disease

Lifestyle modifications play a pivotal role in the comprehensive management of carotid artery disease, specifically carotid artery stenosis. These modifications aim to address risk factors, promote vascular health, and reduce the progression of atherosclerosis. Implementing positive lifestyle changes is essential for both primary prevention and as an adjunct to medical and interventional therapies. The following sections outline key lifestyle modifications in the management of carotid artery disease.

Dietary Interventions

1. **Heart-Healthy Diet:**
    - **Emphasis on Fruits and Vegetables:** A diet rich in fruits and vegetables provides essential vitamins, minerals, and antioxidants, contributing to overall cardiovascular health.
    - **Whole Grains:** Choosing whole grains over refined carbohydrates supports better blood sugar control and provides sustained energy.

2. **Low-Fat and Low-Cholesterol Diet:**
   - **Reducing Saturated and Trans Fats:** Limiting saturated and trans fats helps lower LDL cholesterol levels, reducing the risk of atherosclerosis progression.
   - **Healthy Fat Sources:** Incorporating sources of healthy fats, such as omega-3 fatty acids from fatty fish, can have a positive impact on lipid profiles.
3. **Salt Restriction:**
   - **Sodium Reduction:** Limiting salt intake helps manage blood pressure, reducing the strain on arterial walls and promoting vascular health.

Smoking Cessation

1. **Tobacco Abstinence:**
   - **Immediate and Long-Term Benefits:** Quitting smoking leads to immediate improvements in vascular function and a reduction in cardiovascular risk.
   - **Support Programs:** Engaging in smoking cessation programs, counseling, or using nicotine replacement therapies can enhance the likelihood of successful quitting.

Regular Physical Activity

1. **Aerobic Exercise:**
   - **Cardiovascular Benefits:** Regular aerobic exercise, such as brisk walking, cycling, or swimming, improves cardiovascular fitness and helps control weight.
   - **Frequency and Duration:** Aim for at least 150 minutes of moderate-intensity aerobic exercise

per week, as recommended by health guidelines.
2. **Strength Training:**
   - **Muscle Health:** Incorporating strength training exercises enhances muscle tone, metabolism, and overall physical function.
   - **Balanced Exercise Routine:** Combining aerobic and strength training activities ensures a well-rounded fitness regimen.

Weight Management

1. **Healthy Body Weight:**
   - **Body Mass Index (BMI) Control:** Maintaining a healthy BMI reduces the strain on the cardiovascular system and lowers the risk of obesity-related complications.
   - **Caloric Balance:** Balancing calorie intake with energy expenditure is crucial for weight management.
2. **Waist Circumference:**
   - **Abdominal Obesity Awareness:** Monitoring waist circumference helps identify individuals with abdominal obesity, a risk factor for atherosclerosis.
   - **Targeted Abdominal Exercises:** Incorporating exercises targeting the abdominal muscles can help manage waist circumference.

Blood Pressure Control

1. **Adherence to Medications:**
   - **Antihypertensive Medications:** Consistent use of prescribed antihypertensive medications is essential for controlling blood pressure and preventing further damage to arterial walls.

- **Regular Monitoring:** Regular blood pressure monitoring, both at home and during healthcare visits, facilitates timely adjustments to medication regimens.

2. **Lifestyle Approaches:**
   - **Low-Sodium Diet:** Complementing medication with a low-sodium diet supports blood pressure management.
   - **Stress Reduction Techniques:** Engaging in stress-reducing activities, such as mindfulness, meditation, or yoga, contributes to overall cardiovascular well-being.

Diabetes Management

1. **Blood Glucose Control:**
   - **Adherence to Medications and Insulin:** Managing diabetes through consistent medication adherence and insulin use helps prevent vascular complications.
   - **Blood Sugar Monitoring:** Regular blood glucose monitoring assists in maintaining optimal levels and preventing fluctuations.
2. **Lifestyle Choices:**
   - **Healthy Eating:** Following a diabetes-friendly diet with controlled carbohydrate intake promotes stable blood sugar levels.
   - **Physical Activity:** Regular exercise aids in glucose control and enhances insulin sensitivity.

Stress Reduction and Mental Well-Being

1. **Stress Management Techniques:**
   - **Mindfulness and Relaxation:** Incorporating mindfulness practices, deep breathing exercises,

or relaxation techniques helps reduce stress and promotes vascular health.
- **Counseling or Therapy:** Seeking professional counseling or therapy can provide valuable support in managing stress and maintaining mental well-being.

2. **Adequate Sleep:**
   - **Sleep Hygiene Practices:** Establishing good sleep hygiene, including consistent sleep patterns and a comfortable sleep environment, contributes to overall health.
   - **Addressing Sleep Disorders:** Treating sleep disorders, such as sleep apnea, is crucial for cardiovascular health.

Moderate Alcohol Consumption

1. **Limiting Alcohol Intake:**
   - **Moderation is Key:** If alcohol is consumed, moderation is advised. Limiting intake to moderate levels can have potential cardiovascular benefits.
   - **Individual Considerations:** Factors such as age, health status, and medication interactions should be considered when determining an individual's appropriate alcohol consumption.

Medication Adherence

1. **Compliance with Prescribed Medications:**
   - **Antiplatelet Therapy:** Adhering to prescribed antiplatelet medications, such as aspirin, is essential for preventing blood clot formation in narrowed arteries.
   - **Cholesterol-Lowering Medications:** Consistent use of statins and other lipid-lowering

medications helps control cholesterol levels and stabilize plaques.
2. **Regular Medical Follow-Up:**
    - **Monitoring and Adjustments:** Regular follow-up with healthcare providers allows for monitoring of disease progression and adjustments to the treatment plan as needed.

Implementing these lifestyle modifications requires a multidisciplinary approach involving healthcare providers, nutritionists, physical therapists, and mental health professionals. Patient education, ongoing support, and the cultivation of sustainable habits are key components of successful lifestyle interventions in the management of carotid artery disease. Tailoring recommendations to individual needs and preferences enhances the likelihood of long-term adherence and positive outcomes.

Pharmacotherapy in the Management of Carotid Artery Disease

Pharmacotherapy plays a crucial role in the comprehensive management of carotid artery disease, particularly carotid artery stenosis. The utilization of medications is aimed at addressing specific risk factors, preventing complications, and slowing the progression of atherosclerosis. In this section, we delve into the pharmacological interventions commonly employed in the management of carotid artery disease.

Antiplatelet Agents

1. **Aspirin (Acetylsalicylic Acid):**
    - **Mechanism of Action:** Aspirin inhibits the activity of platelets by irreversibly acetylating

cyclooxygenase (COX), thereby reducing the production of thromboxane A2, a potent platelet aggregator.
- **Primary Prevention:** Aspirin is often prescribed for primary prevention in individuals at high risk for cardiovascular events, including those with carotid artery disease.
- **Secondary Prevention:** In patients with established carotid artery disease or a history of stroke, aspirin is a cornerstone of secondary prevention, significantly reducing the risk of recurrent events.

2. **Clopidogrel and Dual Antiplatelet Therapy:**
   - **Mechanism of Action:** Clopidogrel is an adenosine diphosphate (ADP) receptor antagonist that inhibits platelet aggregation. Dual antiplatelet therapy, combining aspirin and clopidogrel, may be recommended in specific cases.
   - **Post-Carotid Intervention:** Following carotid endarterectomy or stenting, dual antiplatelet therapy is often prescribed to prevent thrombotic complications.

3. **Ticagrelor and Prasugrel:**
   - **Alternative Antiplatelet Agents:** Ticagrelor and prasugrel are newer antiplatelet agents that may be considered in certain situations, particularly in patients with acute coronary syndromes.

4. **Cilostazol:**
   - **Phosphodiesterase Inhibitor:** Cilostazol inhibits phosphodiesterase III, leading to increased cyclic adenosine monophosphate (cAMP) levels, which ultimately inhibits platelet aggregation and promotes vasodilation.

- **Intermittent Claudication:** Cilostazol is approved for the treatment of intermittent claudication in peripheral artery disease and may be considered in patients with carotid artery disease.

Lipid-Lowering Drugs

1. **Statins:**
    - **Mechanism of Action:** Statins, such as atorvastatin and simvastatin, inhibit HMG-CoA reductase, a key enzyme in cholesterol synthesis. By lowering LDL cholesterol levels, statins have anti-inflammatory and plaque-stabilizing effects.
    - **Primary and Secondary Prevention:** Statins are a cornerstone in the management of carotid artery disease, both for primary prevention in high-risk individuals and secondary prevention in those with established disease.
    - **High-Intensity Statin Therapy:** In cases of severe carotid artery stenosis or a history of cardiovascular events, high-intensity statin therapy is often recommended to achieve optimal lipid control.
2. **Ezetimibe:**
    - **Cholesterol Absorption Inhibitor:** Ezetimibe inhibits the absorption of cholesterol in the small intestine, leading to reduced LDL cholesterol levels.
    - **Combination Therapy:** Ezetimibe may be prescribed as an adjunct to statin therapy to achieve additional LDL cholesterol lowering, especially in cases where statins alone are insufficient or not tolerated.
3. **PCSK9 Inhibitors (Alirocumab, Evolocumab):**
    - **Mechanism of Action:** PCSK9 inhibitors block the

action of proprotein convertase subtilisin/kexin type 9 (PCSK9), increasing the number of hepatic LDL receptors and enhancing LDL cholesterol clearance from the bloodstream.
- **Adjunct Therapy:** PCSK9 inhibitors are considered in cases where maximal tolerated statin therapy does not achieve target LDL cholesterol levels.

4. **Bile Acid Sequestrants:**
   - **Cholesterol Binding Agents:** Bile acid sequestrants, such as cholestyramine, bind to bile acids in the intestine, leading to increased excretion of cholesterol and reduced LDL cholesterol levels.
   - **Considerations and Side Effects:** While effective, these agents are less commonly used due to gastrointestinal side effects and potential interactions with other medications.

Antihypertensive Medications

1. **Angiotensin-Converting Enzyme (ACE) Inhibitors:**
   - **Mechanism of Action:** ACE inhibitors, like enalapril and lisinopril, inhibit the conversion of angiotensin I to angiotensin II, leading to vasodilation and reduced aldosterone secretion.
   - **Vasoprotective Effects:** ACE inhibitors have vasoprotective effects, preserving endothelial function and reducing vascular inflammation.
   - **Indications:** ACE inhibitors are commonly prescribed for hypertension management and may be beneficial in individuals with carotid artery disease, particularly if there are concurrent cardiovascular risk factors.
2. **Angiotensin II Receptor Blockers (ARBs):**

- **Mechanism of Action:** ARBs, such as losartan and valsartan, block the action of angiotensin II at its receptors, leading to vasodilation and reduced aldosterone secretion.
- **Alternative to ACE Inhibitors:** In cases where ACE inhibitors are not well-tolerated, ARBs are considered as an alternative for blood pressure control and vasoprotection.

3. **Calcium Channel Blockers:**
   - **Mechanism of Action:** Calcium channel blockers, including amlodipine and nifedipine, block calcium entry into vascular smooth muscle cells, leading to vasodilation.
   - **Blood Pressure Control:** Calcium channel blockers are effective in managing hypertension and may be prescribed as part of antihypertensive therapy in individuals with carotid artery disease.

4. **Beta-Blockers:**
   - **Mechanism of Action:** Beta-blockers, such as metoprolol and carvedilol, reduce heart rate and blood pressure by blocking the effects of catecholamines on beta receptors.
   - **Heart Rate Control:** Beta-blockers are indicated in specific cases to control heart rate, particularly in individuals with concurrent coronary artery disease or atrial fibrillation.

5. **Thiazide Diuretics:**
   - **Mechanism of Action:** Thiazide diuretics, like hydrochlorothiazide, promote diuresis and reduce blood volume, leading to decreased blood pressure.
   - **Combination Therapy:** Thiazide diuretics are often used in combination with other antihypertensive agents to achieve optimal blood pressure control.

6. **Diuretics:**
   - **Fluid and Sodium Balance:** Diuretics, including loop diuretics like furosemide, help regulate fluid and sodium balance, contributing to blood pressure control.
   - **Edema Management:** In cases of concomitant heart failure or edema, diuretics may be prescribed to alleviate fluid retention.

Medication Combinations and Individualization

1. **Combination Therapy:**
   - **Polypharmacy Considerations:** In some cases, combination therapy involving multiple classes of antihypertensive medications or a combination of antiplatelet and lipid-lowering agents may be warranted.
   - **Individualized Approach:** Medication regimens are tailored to individual patient characteristics, including age, comorbidities, and tolerability.
2. **Risk-Benefit Assessment:**
   - **Shared Decision-Making:** Shared decision-making between healthcare providers and patients involves discussing the potential benefits and risks of pharmacotherapy, considering individual circumstances.
   - **Monitoring and Adjustments:** Regular monitoring of medication efficacy and potential side effects allows for timely adjustments to optimize treatment outcomes.
3. **Adherence and Follow-Up:**
   - **Patient Education:** Providing comprehensive patient education on the importance of medication adherence, potential side effects, and the overall management plan fosters patient

engagement.
- **Regular Follow-Up:** Scheduled follow-up appointments enable healthcare providers to assess treatment response, address concerns, and make necessary adjustments.

Emerging Therapies and Research Directions

1. **Innovations in Antiplatelet Therapy:**
   - **Novel Antiplatelet Agents:** Ongoing research is exploring the development of novel antiplatelet agents with improved efficacy and safety profiles.
   - **Personalized Antiplatelet Therapy:** Advancements in genetic testing may contribute to personalized antiplatelet therapy, tailoring treatment based on an individual's genetic response.
2. **Advanced Lipid-Lowering Strategies:**
   - **RNA-Based Therapies:** Investigational RNA-based therapies, such as RNA interference (RNAi) targeting specific genes, show promise in achieving precise control of lipid metabolism.
   - **Precision Medicine Approaches:** Precision medicine approaches aim to identify genetic markers influencing lipid response to inform personalized lipid-lowering strategies.
3. **Targeted Antihypertensive Therapies:**
   - **Renal Denervation:** Renal denervation, a procedure targeting renal sympathetic nerves, is under investigation as a potential therapeutic approach for resistant hypertension.
   - **Renin-Angiotensin System Modulation:** Ongoing research explores novel agents targeting components of the renin-angiotensin system for more effective blood pressure control.

4. **Combinatorial Approaches:**
    - **Multimodal Therapy:** Investigational studies are exploring the effectiveness of combining multiple pharmacotherapeutic agents, addressing various aspects of atherosclerosis and cardiovascular risk.
    - **Interdisciplinary Collaboration:** Collaboration between cardiology, neurology, and vascular medicine specialists is crucial for implementing comprehensive, multidisciplinary approaches.

Pharmacotherapy in carotid artery disease management is a dynamic and evolving field, with ongoing research aimed at improving treatment outcomes and tailoring interventions to individual patient needs. The integration of emerging therapies, precision medicine approaches, and a focus on combinatorial strategies underscores the commitment to advancing patient care in the realm of carotid artery disease. Regular updates in clinical guidelines reflect the evolving evidence base, ensuring that healthcare providers can offer the most effective and personalized pharmacotherapeutic interventions to individuals with carotid artery disease.

Dietary Recommendations in the Management of Carotid Artery Disease

Diet plays a fundamental role in the management of carotid artery disease, influencing key risk factors such as cholesterol levels, blood pressure, and overall vascular health. Adopting a heart-healthy diet can contribute significantly to the prevention of atherosclerosis progression and reduce the risk of complications. The following dietary recommendations are tailored to individuals with carotid artery disease, focusing on optimizing cardiovascular health and supporting overall well-being.

Heart-Healthy Dietary Patterns

1. **Mediterranean Diet:**
   - **Emphasis on Plant-Based Foods:** The Mediterranean diet places a strong emphasis on fruits, vegetables, whole grains, nuts, and legumes, providing essential vitamins, minerals, and antioxidants.
   - **Healthy Fats:** Incorporating olive oil as the primary source of dietary fat contributes monounsaturated fats, which have been associated with cardiovascular benefits.
2. **DASH Diet (Dietary Approaches to Stop Hypertension):**
   - **Sodium Restriction:** The DASH diet emphasizes reducing sodium intake, promoting the consumption of fresh fruits, vegetables, and lean proteins.
   - **Calcium and Potassium-Rich Foods:** High intake of calcium and potassium-rich foods, such as dairy products, nuts, and bananas, supports blood pressure control.
3. **Plant-Based Diet:**
   - **Reduced Animal Products:** A plant-based diet limits the intake of red and processed meats, emphasizing plant-derived proteins such as beans, lentils, and tofu.
   - **Omega-3 Fatty Acids:** Including sources of omega-3 fatty acids, such as flaxseeds, chia seeds, and fatty fish, contributes to anti-inflammatory effects.

Nutrient-Specific Recommendations

1. **Cholesterol-Lowering Foods:**

- **Soluble Fiber Sources:** Foods rich in soluble fiber, including oats, barley, and legumes, help reduce LDL cholesterol levels.
- **Plant Sterols and Stanols:** Incorporating foods fortified with plant sterols and stanols, such as certain margarines, supports cholesterol reduction.

2. **Omega-3 Fatty Acids:**
   - **Fatty Fish:** Consuming fatty fish, such as salmon, mackerel, and trout, provides omega-3 fatty acids, which have anti-inflammatory and cardiovascular benefits.
   - **Plant-Based Sources:** Including plant-based sources of omega-3s, like walnuts, flaxseeds, and chia seeds, is beneficial for individuals with dietary restrictions.

3. **Antioxidant-Rich Foods:**
   - **Colorful Fruits and Vegetables:** Consuming a variety of colorful fruits and vegetables ensures a diverse intake of antioxidants, protecting against oxidative stress.
   - **Berries:** Berries, such as blueberries and strawberries, are rich in antioxidants and may have specific cardiovascular benefits.

4. **Whole Grains:**
   - **Brown Rice, Quinoa, and Whole Wheat:** Choosing whole grains over refined grains provides fiber, vitamins, and minerals, contributing to overall cardiovascular health.
   - **Fiber-Rich Cereals:** Opting for cereals high in fiber without added sugars supports satiety and helps regulate blood sugar levels.

5. **Low-Fat Dairy or Dairy Alternatives:**
   - **Calcium and Vitamin D:** Incorporating low-

fat dairy or fortified dairy alternatives ensures an adequate intake of calcium and vitamin D, essential for bone health.
- **Moderation is Key:** Choosing low-fat options helps manage saturated fat intake while maintaining essential nutrients.

3 Dietary Restrictions and Considerations

1. **Sodium Restriction:**
   - **Fresh Foods:** Choosing fresh, unprocessed foods and minimizing the use of added salt during cooking and at the table supports sodium restriction.
   - **Herbs and Spices:** Utilizing herbs, spices, and other flavorings as alternatives to salt enhances the taste of dishes without compromising dietary goals.
2. **Limiting Saturated and Trans Fats:**
   - **Lean Protein Sources:** Opting for lean protein sources, such as skinless poultry, fish, and plant-based proteins, helps limit saturated fat intake.
   - **Trans Fat Avoidance:** Avoiding processed and fried foods containing trans fats is crucial for cardiovascular health.
3. **Moderation in Added Sugars:**
   - **Natural Sweeteners:** Choosing natural sweeteners like honey or maple syrup in moderation instead of refined sugars supports a heart-healthy diet.
   - **Reading Labels:** Checking food labels for hidden sugars and opting for minimally processed options helps reduce added sugar intake.
4. **Individualized Caloric Intake:**
   - **Maintaining Healthy Weight:** Adjusting caloric intake based on individual energy needs and

maintaining a healthy weight is integral to cardiovascular health.
- **Professional Guidance:** Seeking guidance from a registered dietitian or healthcare provider ensures individualized nutritional recommendations.

Hydration and Beverage Choices

1. **Water Intake:**
   - **Adequate Hydration:** Drinking an adequate amount of water throughout the day supports overall health and hydration, contributing to optimal vascular function.
   - **Limiting Sugary Beverages:** Reducing the consumption of sugary drinks and opting for water or unsweetened herbal teas promotes a healthier beverage choice.
2. **Limiting Alcohol Intake:**
   - **Moderation is Key:** If alcohol is consumed, moderation is advised. For individuals with carotid artery disease, limiting alcohol intake to moderate levels is generally recommended.
   - **Individual Considerations:** Factors such as age, health status, and potential interactions with medications should be considered.

Practical Tips for Implementation

1. **Meal Planning and Preparation:**
   - **Batch Cooking:** Preparing meals in batches and incorporating a variety of nutrient-dense ingredients simplifies meal planning and supports dietary goals.
   - **Incorporating Diversity:** Including a diverse range of foods ensures a broad spectrum of nutrients, contributing to overall nutritional well-

being.
2. **Education and Awareness:**
   - **Nutritional Label Reading:** Developing the habit of reading nutritional labels helps individuals make informed choices and monitor their intake of key nutrients.
   - **Educational Resources:** Accessing educational resources on heart-healthy eating, such as dietary guidelines and reputable websites, enhances nutritional literacy.
3. **Culinary Techniques:**
   - **Healthy Cooking Methods:** Utilizing healthy cooking methods, such as grilling, steaming, or roasting, preserves nutritional content while minimizing added fats.
   - **Herbs and Spices:** Experimenting with herbs and spices enhances the flavor of dishes without relying on excessive salt or unhealthy condiments.
4. **Mindful Eating:**
   - **Savoring Meals:** Practicing mindful eating, savoring each bite and paying attention to hunger and fullness cues, promotes a healthy relationship with food.
   - **Avoiding Distractions:** Minimizing distractions during meals, such as electronic devices, encourages mindful eating and appreciation of food.
5. **Regular Monitoring:**
   - **Food Diary:** Keeping a food diary can aid in tracking dietary habits, identifying patterns, and making necessary adjustments.
   - **Periodic Review:** Periodic review with a registered dietitian or healthcare provider allows for ongoing assessment and refinement of dietary

strategies.

Adhering to heart-healthy dietary recommendations is a pivotal aspect of the multifaceted approach to managing carotid artery disease. While dietary modifications alone may not replace medical interventions, they significantly contribute to the overall cardiovascular health of individuals with carotid artery disease. Empowering individuals with the knowledge and tools to make informed dietary choices fosters a proactive role in their health and well-being, aligning with the broader goal of preventing disease progression and optimizing long-term outcomes.

Smoking Cessation in Carotid Artery Disease Management

Smoking cessation is a critical component of the comprehensive approach to managing carotid artery disease, specifically carotid artery stenosis. Cigarette smoking is a major modifiable risk factor for the development and progression of atherosclerosis, contributing to arterial inflammation, endothelial dysfunction, and the formation of atherosclerotic plaques. This section explores the importance of smoking cessation, the impact of smoking on carotid artery disease, and strategies for individuals to quit smoking.

The Impact of Smoking on Carotid Artery Disease

1. **Endothelial Dysfunction:**
   - **Vasoconstriction:** Smoking leads to the release of vasoconstrictive substances, reducing blood flow and promoting endothelial dysfunction in the carotid arteries.
   - **Impaired Nitric Oxide Production:** Nitric oxide, a crucial vasodilator, is impaired by smoking, compromising the ability of arteries to dilate and

respond to increased demand.
2. **Inflammation and Atherosclerosis:**
   - **Inflammatory Mediators:** Smoking triggers the release of inflammatory mediators, enhancing the inflammatory response in the arterial walls.
   - **Accelerated Atherosclerosis:** Chronic exposure to tobacco smoke accelerates the progression of atherosclerosis, leading to the formation of plaques in the carotid arteries.
3. **Increased Blood Clotting:**
   - **Platelet Aggregation:** Smoking promotes platelet aggregation, increasing the risk of thrombus formation in the carotid arteries.
   - **Prothrombotic State:** The prothrombotic state induced by smoking heightens the likelihood of blood clot formation within narrowed or diseased segments of the carotid arteries.
4. **Impact on Lipid Profile:**
   - **Altered Lipid Metabolism:** Smoking is associated with alterations in lipid metabolism, including decreased levels of high-density lipoprotein (HDL) cholesterol.
   - **Unfavorable Lipid Ratios:** Individuals who smoke often exhibit unfavorable lipid profiles, contributing to the atherosclerotic process in the carotid arteries.

Benefits of Smoking Cessation

1. **Rapid Cardiovascular Improvements:**
   - **Immediate Benefits:** The cardiovascular system begins to show improvements shortly after quitting smoking, with increased oxygen delivery and reduced stress on the carotid arteries.
   - **Blood Pressure Reduction:** Quitting smoking

leads to a decrease in blood pressure, alleviating strain on the arterial walls.

2. **Reduction in Atherosclerosis Progression:**
   - **Slowing Plaque Formation:** Smoking cessation slows the progression of atherosclerosis, reducing the likelihood of further narrowing in the carotid arteries.
   - **Stabilization of Plaques:** The risk of plaque rupture, a critical event leading to thrombus formation, decreases with sustained smoking cessation.

3. **Improved Endothelial Function:**
   - **Enhanced Vasodilation:** Quitting smoking contributes to improved endothelial function, allowing for better vasodilation and blood flow in the carotid arteries.
   - **Preservation of Nitric Oxide:** The restoration of nitric oxide production supports the health of the endothelium and vascular function.

4. **Positive Effects on Lipid Profile:**
   - **Increased HDL Cholesterol:** Smoking cessation is associated with an increase in HDL cholesterol levels, contributing to a more favorable lipid profile.
   - **Lipid Stabilization:** The lipid profile stabilizes with cessation, reducing the proatherogenic effects associated with smoking.

Strategies for Smoking Cessation

1. **Behavioral Support Programs:**
   - **Counseling Services:** Behavioral counseling, either individually or in group settings, provides support for individuals attempting to quit smoking.

- **Cognitive-Behavioral Therapy (CBT):** CBT techniques help individuals identify and manage triggers for smoking, fostering sustainable behavioral changes.

2. **Pharmacotherapy:**
   - **Nicotine Replacement Therapy (NRT):** NRT, including patches, gum, lozenges, nasal spray, and inhalers, provides controlled doses of nicotine to help manage withdrawal symptoms.
   - **Prescription Medications:** Medications such as bupropion and varenicline may be prescribed to aid in smoking cessation by reducing cravings and withdrawal symptoms.

3. **Mobile Applications and Online Resources:**
   - **Quitline Services:** Many countries offer quitline services with trained professionals providing support and guidance.
   - **Mobile Apps:** Smartphone applications designed for smoking cessation offer interactive tools, progress tracking, and motivational support.

4. **Support from Healthcare Providers:**
   - **Individualized Plans:** Healthcare providers collaborate with individuals to develop personalized smoking cessation plans, considering medical history, preferences, and potential challenges.
   - **Regular Follow-Up:** Scheduled follow-up appointments allow healthcare providers to monitor progress, address concerns, and make necessary adjustments to the cessation plan.

5. **Social Support and Peer Groups:**
   - **Supportive Networks:** Engaging with friends, family, or support groups provides a crucial network for encouragement and accountability.

- **Peer Experiences:** Sharing experiences with individuals who have successfully quit smoking can be motivating and inspiring for those on their cessation journey.

6. **Stress Management Techniques:**
   - **Alternative Coping Strategies:** Identifying alternative coping strategies for stress, such as mindfulness, meditation, or physical activity, helps reduce reliance on smoking as a stress reliever.
   - **Integrated Approaches:** Combining stress management techniques with smoking cessation efforts enhances overall well-being.

7. **Educational Initiatives:**
   - **Understanding Health Risks:** Education on the specific health risks associated with smoking and the benefits of quitting fosters motivation.
   - **Long-Term Health Perspectives:** Emphasizing the long-term positive effects of smoking cessation on cardiovascular health and overall well-being is integral to sustained motivation.

Smoking cessation is a transformative step towards improving cardiovascular health and mitigating the progression of carotid artery disease. The integration of evidence-based strategies, ongoing support, and a multidisciplinary approach involving healthcare providers, behavioral specialists, and support networks significantly enhances the likelihood of successful smoking cessation. Recognizing the profound impact of quitting smoking on arterial health underscores the importance of prioritizing smoking cessation as a fundamental component of carotid artery disease management.

CHAPTER 8: SURGICAL INTERVENTIONS

Carotid Endarterectomy (CEA) in the Management of Carotid Artery Disease

Carotid endarterectomy (CEA) is a surgical procedure designed to treat carotid artery disease, specifically carotid artery stenosis. This intervention is aimed at reducing the risk of stroke by removing atherosclerotic plaque from the carotid arteries, thus improving blood flow to the brain. This section provides a comprehensive exploration of carotid endarterectomy, encompassing its indications, contraindications, and various procedural techniques.

Indications and Contraindications

Indications for Carotid Endarterectomy (CEA):

1. **Symptomatic Carotid Artery Stenosis:**
    - Individuals who have experienced a transient ischemic attack (TIA) or minor stroke related to significant carotid artery stenosis may be candidates for CEA.
    - Symptomatic patients with moderate to severe carotid artery stenosis are considered for the procedure to reduce the risk of recurrent

cerebrovascular events.
2. **Asymptomatic High-Grade Carotid Stenosis:**
    - Asymptomatic individuals with high-grade carotid artery stenosis, typically exceeding 70%, may be considered for CEA, particularly if they belong to high-risk groups for future cerebrovascular events.
3. **Progressive Symptoms despite Medical Therapy:**
    - Patients who continue to experience neurological symptoms despite optimal medical management, including antiplatelet therapy and statins, may be evaluated for carotid endarterectomy.
4. **High-Grade Stenosis with Significant Life Expectancy:**
    - In asymptomatic individuals with a significant life expectancy and high-grade carotid artery stenosis, the potential long-term benefits of preventing stroke may outweigh the risks associated with the procedure.
5. **Combined Carotid and Coronary Artery Disease:**
    - Patients with concomitant carotid and coronary artery disease may be considered for carotid endarterectomy, especially when coronary artery bypass grafting (CABG) is planned.

Contraindications to Carotid Endarterectomy (CEA):

1. **High Surgical Risk:**
    - Patients with a high surgical risk due to comorbidities, such as severe heart failure, advanced age, or significant pulmonary disease, may be deemed unsuitable candidates for carotid endarterectomy.
2. **Severe Neurological Impairment:**
    - Individuals with severe neurological impairment, including large strokes with extensive brain

damage, may not benefit from carotid endarterectomy, as the procedure aims to prevent future events rather than reverse existing neurological deficits.

3. **Unstable Medical Conditions:**
   - Unstable medical conditions, such as uncontrolled hypertension, recent myocardial infarction, or active infections, may preclude individuals from undergoing elective surgery.

4. **Inaccessible Carotid Lesions:**
   - Carotid lesions that are inaccessible or challenging to reach surgically may present contraindications to carotid endarterectomy.

5. **Unfavorable Anatomy:**
   - Unfavorable carotid artery anatomy, such as excessive tortuosity or calcification, may pose challenges during the surgical procedure and influence the decision to perform carotid endarterectomy.

6. **Patient Refusal:**
   - In cases where patients actively refuse the procedure, their autonomy and preferences should be respected, and alternative management options should be explored.

Procedure Techniques

Preoperative Evaluation:

1. **Clinical Assessment:**
   - A thorough clinical assessment is conducted, including a detailed neurological examination, assessment of risk factors, and evaluation of the patient's overall health.

2. **Imaging Studies:**
   - Non-invasive imaging studies, such as carotid

ultrasound, magnetic resonance angiography (MRA), or computed tomography angiography (CTA), provide detailed information about the extent and severity of carotid artery stenosis.

3. **Cerebral Blood Flow Assessment:**
   - Assessment of cerebral blood flow using techniques like transcranial Doppler ultrasound helps evaluate the adequacy of collateral circulation and guides decision-making.

4. **Cardiac Evaluation:**
   - Cardiac evaluation, including electrocardiogram (ECG) and echocardiography, is performed to assess the patient's cardiac status and identify any coexisting cardiovascular conditions.

5. **Risk Stratification:**
   - Risk stratification is crucial to determine the patient's suitability for carotid endarterectomy. This involves evaluating the overall surgical risk based on comorbidities, age, and the extent of carotid artery disease.

Surgical Technique:

1. **Anesthesia:**
   - Carotid endarterectomy is typically performed under regional anesthesia, such as cervical plexus block or carotid artery block, allowing for continuous neurological monitoring during the procedure.

2. **Access and Exposure:**
   - A small incision is made in the neck over the affected carotid artery, providing access to the arterial segment with stenosis. The surgeon carefully exposes and isolates the carotid artery.

3. **Arteriotomy:**

- An arteriotomy is made in the carotid artery, usually longitudinally, exposing the atherosclerotic plaque. The surgeon must handle the artery with care to minimize the risk of embolization.

4. **Endarterectomy:**
   - The atherosclerotic plaque is carefully dissected and removed from the arterial wall, restoring normal blood flow. The surgeon may use specialized shunts to maintain cerebral perfusion during plaque removal.

5. **Closure of Arteriotomy:**
   - The arteriotomy is closed with a patch, which may be an autologous vessel (e.g., saphenous vein) or synthetic material. The choice of patch depends on factors such as vessel size and surgeon preference.

6. **Hemostasis:**
   - Hemostasis is crucial to prevent postoperative bleeding. The surgeon ensures that the artery is free of clots or debris before closing the incision.

7. **Closure of Incision:**
   - The neck incision is closed with sutures, and a sterile dressing is applied. The patient is monitored closely in the immediate postoperative period for any signs of complications.

Postoperative Care:

1. **Neurological Monitoring:**
   - Continuous neurological monitoring is maintained postoperatively to detect any signs of stroke or complications promptly.

2. **Blood Pressure Management:**
   - Blood pressure is carefully managed to optimize

cerebral perfusion while minimizing the risk of hyperperfusion syndrome or bleeding at the surgical site.

3. **Antithrombotic Therapy:**
   - Antithrombotic therapy, often initiated preoperatively, is continued postoperatively to prevent thrombus formation and promote graft patency.

4. **Early Mobilization:**
   - Early mobilization is encouraged to prevent complications such as deep vein thrombosis and aid in overall recovery.

5. **Monitoring for Complications:**
   - Close monitoring for complications, including hematoma, infection, or neurological deficits, is essential during the initial recovery period.

6. **Follow-Up Imaging:**
   - Follow-up imaging studies, such as carotid ultrasound or angiography, may be performed to assess the success of the procedure and the patency of the carotid artery.

7. **Long-Term Follow-Up:**
   - Long-term follow-up involves ongoing surveillance of the patient's carotid artery disease, neurological status, and overall cardiovascular health to ensure optimal outcomes.

Advances and Innovations in CEA:

1. **Minimally Invasive Techniques:**
   - Some centers are exploring minimally invasive techniques for carotid endarterectomy, including endovascular approaches and robotic-assisted surgery. These techniques aim to reduce surgical trauma and enhance recovery.

2. **Patchless Endarterectomy:**
   - Patchless endarterectomy, where the arteriotomy is closed primarily without using a patch, is being investigated as an alternative approach. Studies are ongoing to evaluate the long-term outcomes and safety of this technique.
3. **Hybrid Procedures:**
   - Hybrid procedures, combining carotid endarterectomy with concurrent coronary artery bypass grafting or other cardiovascular interventions, may be considered in selected cases to address multiple arterial issues simultaneously.
4. **Role of Imaging in Surgical Planning:**
   - Advances in preoperative imaging, such as three-dimensional reconstructions and virtual surgical planning, contribute to more precise surgical interventions and personalized approaches.

Conclusion:

Carotid endarterectomy remains a cornerstone in the management of carotid artery disease, offering a targeted and effective intervention to reduce the risk of stroke in selected patients. The careful selection of candidates based on comprehensive preoperative evaluation, including clinical, imaging, and cardiac assessments, is essential to ensure favorable outcomes. Advances in surgical techniques, perioperative care, and ongoing research contribute to refining the approach to carotid endarterectomy, with a focus on improving patient safety and long-term results.

As the field of vascular surgery continues to evolve, ongoing research endeavors and technological innovations will likely shape the future landscape of carotid endarterectomy. The integration of evidence-based practices, adherence to guidelines, and a commitment to individualized patient care collectively contribute to the ongoing success of carotid endarterectomy as a crucial intervention in the comprehensive management of carotid artery disease.

Carotid Artery Stenting (CAS) in the Management of Carotid Artery Disease

Carotid artery stenting (CAS) has emerged as an alternative to carotid endarterectomy (CEA) in the management of carotid artery disease, particularly carotid artery stenosis. This section provides a comprehensive exploration of carotid artery stenting, covering aspects such as patient selection, procedural considerations, and the evolving landscape of this endovascular intervention.

Patient Selection

Indications for Carotid Artery Stenting (CAS):

1. **Symptomatic Carotid Artery Stenosis:**
   - CAS is indicated for individuals with symptomatic carotid artery stenosis who are considered high surgical risk or have anatomical considerations that make carotid endarterectomy (CEA) challenging.
2. **Asymptomatic High-Grade Stenosis:**
   - Asymptomatic patients with high-grade carotid artery stenosis, particularly those deemed high risk for CEA, may be considered for CAS based on individualized risk-benefit assessments.
3. **Concomitant Coronary or Aortic Disease:**
   - Patients with carotid artery disease who also have significant coronary artery disease or aortic pathology may benefit from a simultaneous or

staged intervention, making CAS a viable option.

4. **High-Risk Surgical Candidates:**
   - Individuals deemed high risk for surgery due to comorbidities such as advanced age, severe heart or lung disease, or previous neck surgery may be suitable candidates for CAS.

5. **Anatomical Considerations:**
   - Anatomical factors, such as the presence of extensive scarring from previous surgeries, high carotid bifurcation, or contralateral carotid occlusion, may favor CAS as a preferred intervention.

6. **Patient Preference:**
   - In shared decision-making, patient preference plays a crucial role. Some individuals may prefer an endovascular approach, and their values and preferences should be considered in the decision-making process.

Contraindications to Carotid Artery Stenting (CAS):

1. **Accessible Carotid Lesions:**
   - Lesions that are inaccessible or challenging to reach with endovascular techniques may be considered contraindications to CAS.

2. **Unstable Medical Conditions:**
   - Patients with unstable medical conditions, such as recent myocardial infarction, uncontrolled hypertension, or active infections, may be contraindicated for elective endovascular procedures.

3. **Severe Renal Impairment:**
   - Severe renal impairment or contraindications to the use of contrast media may limit the feasibility of CAS.

4. **Inability to Tolerate Dual Antiplatelet Therapy:**
   - Individuals unable to tolerate dual antiplatelet therapy, a standard regimen after CAS, due to bleeding disorders or other contraindications, may not be suitable candidates.
5. **Acute Stroke or Transient Ischemic Attack (TIA):**
   - Recent acute stroke or TIA may be a contraindication to elective CAS. In such cases, urgent evaluation and management may be warranted, but the optimal timing of intervention require careful consideration.

Procedural Considerations

Preoperative Evaluation:

1. **Clinical Assessment:**
   - A comprehensive clinical assessment, including a detailed neurological examination and evaluation of cardiovascular risk factors, is conducted to inform the decision-making process.
2. **Imaging Studies:**
   - Non-invasive imaging studies, such as carotid ultrasound, magnetic resonance angiography (MRA), or computed tomography angiography (CTA), provide detailed information about the location and severity of carotid artery stenosis.
3. **Cerebral Blood Flow Assessment:**
   - Assessment of cerebral blood flow using techniques like transcranial Doppler ultrasound helps evaluate the adequacy of collateral circulation and guide procedural planning.
4. **Cardiac Evaluation:**
   - Cardiac evaluation, including electrocardiogram (ECG) and echocardiography, is performed to assess the patient's cardiac status and identify any

coexisting cardiovascular conditions.
5. **Dual Antiplatelet Therapy:**
    - Preoperative initiation of dual antiplatelet therapy, typically with aspirin and clopidogrel, is essential to minimize the risk of thromboembolic events during and after the CAS procedure.

Technical Aspects of Carotid Artery Stenting (CAS):

1. **Access Site:**
    - Access to the carotid artery is typically obtained through the femoral artery using a percutaneous approach. Transradial access is an alternative in selected cases.
2. **Guidewire and Catheter Placement:**
    - A guidewire is navigated through the femoral access to the carotid artery under fluoroscopic guidance. A catheter is then advanced over the guidewire to the site of stenosis.
3. **Angiography and Lesion Assessment:**
    - Contrast angiography is performed to visualize the carotid artery and precisely assess the location and severity of the stenosis. Lesion characteristics, such as calcification or ulceration, are evaluated.
4. **Balloon Angioplasty:**
    - Balloon angioplasty may be employed to dilate the stenotic segment and optimize the vessel diameter before stent placement.
5. **Stent Placement:**
    - A stent, often a self-expanding or balloon-expandable design, is deployed at the site of stenosis to provide mechanical support and prevent vessel recoil. Stent selection depends on the specific characteristics of the lesion.
6. **Distal Protection Devices:**

- Distal protection devices, such as embolic protection filters or balloons, are used to capture debris released during the procedure, reducing the risk of embolic events.

7. **Post-Dilation:**
   - Post-dilation with a balloon may be performed to further optimize stent expansion and apposition to the vessel wall.

8. **Final Angiography:**
   - A final contrast angiography is performed to confirm optimal stent placement, assess blood flow, and detect any residual stenosis or complications.

Postoperative Care:

1. **Neurological Monitoring:**
   - Continuous neurological monitoring is maintained postoperatively to detect any signs of stroke or complications promptly.

2. **Blood Pressure Management:**
   - Blood pressure is carefully managed to optimize cerebral perfusion while minimizing the risk of hyperperfusion syndrome or bleeding at the access site.

3. **Dual Antiplatelet Therapy Continuation:**
   - Dual antiplatelet therapy is continued postoperatively to prevent thromboembolic events and promote stent patency.

4. **Monitoring for Complications:**
   - Close monitoring for complications, including access site issues, embolic events, or neurological deficits, is essential during the initial recovery period.

5. **Follow-Up Imaging:**

- Follow-up imaging studies, such as carotid ultrasound or angiography, may be performed to assess the success of the procedure and the patency of the stented carotid artery.

6. **Long-Term Follow-Up:**
    - Long-term follow-up involves ongoing surveillance of the patient's carotid artery disease, neurological status, and overall cardiovascular health to ensure optimal outcomes.

Evolving Landscape of CAS:

1. **Embolic Protection Devices:**
    - Advances in embolic protection devices aim to enhance procedural safety by minimizing the risk of distal embolization during stent placement.
2. **Stent Design and Materials:**
    - Ongoing research explores novel stent designs and materials, including bioresorbable stents, to improve long-term outcomes and reduce the risk of complications.
3. **Patient-Specific Approaches:**
    - The development of patient-specific treatment algorithms, incorporating factors such as plaque composition, lesion morphology, and individual patient characteristics, contributes to personalized and optimized CAS procedures.
4. **Hybrid Approaches:**
    - Hybrid approaches, combining CAS with other endovascular or surgical interventions, are being explored to address complex cases and provide tailored solutions to patients with multifaceted vascular issues.
5. **Clinical Trials and Research Initiatives:**
    - Ongoing clinical trials and research initiatives

aim to refine the evidence base for CAS, providing valuable insights into the comparative effectiveness, safety, and long-term outcomes of this endovascular intervention.

Conclusion:

Carotid artery stenting (CAS) has established itself as a valuable alternative to carotid endarterectomy (CEA) in selected cases of carotid artery disease, offering a less invasive approach with specific advantages in high-risk surgical candidates. The decision between CAS and CEA requires careful consideration of individual patient characteristics, anatomical factors, and the overall risk-benefit profile. Advances in technology, procedural techniques, and ongoing research continue to shape the landscape of CAS, contributing to improved patient outcomes and expanding the scope of endovascular interventions in the management of carotid artery disease.

As the field of vascular medicine progresses, the integration of evidence-based practices, adherence to guidelines, and ongoing collaboration between interventionalists, vascular surgeons, and multidisciplinary teams remain paramount. The evolution of carotid artery stenting underscores the dynamic nature of vascular interventions, highlighting the importance of staying abreast of emerging technologies and research findings to provide optimal care for individuals with carotid artery disease.

CHAPTER 9: NOVEL THERAPEUTIC APPROACHES

Emerging Pharmacological Therapies in Carotid Artery Disease

Carotid artery disease, characterized by the narrowing or blockage of the carotid arteries, poses a significant risk for stroke and other cardiovascular events. While established treatments such as antiplatelet agents and lipid-lowering drugs play crucial roles in managing this condition, ongoing research is exploring emerging pharmacological therapies to further enhance therapeutic options. This section delves into the latest developments and promising avenues in pharmacotherapy for carotid artery disease.

Novel Antiplatelet Agents:

P2Y12 Receptor Inhibitors:

Recent research has focused on the development of novel P2Y12 receptor inhibitors to augment the antiplatelet armamentarium. These agents target specific pathways involved in platelet activation and aggregation, aiming for enhanced efficacy and reduced bleeding risk compared to traditional antiplatelet medications.

Thromboxane A2 Inhibitors:

Inhibition of thromboxane A2, a potent platelet aggregator, is being explored as a potential strategy to mitigate platelet-driven thrombosis in carotid artery disease. Emerging thromboxane A2 inhibitors may offer a targeted approach to modulating platelet function and preventing thrombotic complications.

Anti-Inflammatory Therapies:

Cytokine Modulators:

Chronic inflammation plays a pivotal role in the progression of atherosclerosis and carotid artery disease. Researchers are investigating cytokine modulators that selectively target inflammatory pathways implicated in plaque development. These agents aim to reduce inflammation within the arterial walls, potentially stabilizing atherosclerotic plaques and lowering the risk of rupture and thrombosis.

Monoclonal Antibodies:

Monoclonal antibodies targeting specific inflammatory markers, such as interleukin-1 beta or tumor necrosis factor-alpha, are being explored for their potential anti-inflammatory effects in carotid artery disease. These biologic agents aim to disrupt inflammatory cascades and may hold promise in attenuating disease progression.

Advanced Lipid-Lowering Therapies:

Proprotein Convertase Subtilisin/Kexin Type 9 (PCSK9) Inhibitors:

PCSK9 inhibitors represent a revolutionary class of drugs that effectively lower low-density lipoprotein (LDL) cholesterol levels by inhibiting the PCSK9 enzyme. These agents, administered either through subcutaneous injections or oral formulations, offer a potent means of achieving LDL cholesterol reduction beyond what is attainable with traditional statin therapy. Ongoing research is exploring the impact of PCSK9 inhibitors on atherosclerosis regression and cardiovascular outcomes in carotid artery disease.

Apolipoprotein B-Targeted Therapies:

Innovative therapies targeting apolipoprotein B, a key component of atherogenic lipoproteins, are under investigation. By specifically addressing apolipoprotein B, these therapies aim to disrupt the formation of atherogenic particles and reduce the burden of lipid deposition in the carotid arteries.

Novel Antithrombotic Approaches:

Factor XI Inhibitors:

Factor XI, a coagulation factor involved in the intrinsic pathway, is under scrutiny as a potential target for antithrombotic therapy. Inhibitors of factor XI are being studied for their ability to modulate thrombotic risk without significantly affecting hemostasis, offering a nuanced approach to preventing thromboembolic events in carotid artery disease.

Direct Oral Anticoagulants (DOACs):

The role of direct oral anticoagulants, traditionally employed in atrial fibrillation and venous thromboembolism, is being explored in the context of carotid artery disease. Studies are investigating the safety and efficacy of DOACs in preventing thromboembolic events in high-risk individuals, providing an alternative to traditional antiplatelet therapy.

Vasoprotective Agents:

Endothelial Function Modulators:

Preserving endothelial function is a critical aspect of

preventing atherosclerosis and maintaining vascular health. Emerging pharmacological agents target endothelial function directly, promoting vasodilation, reducing inflammation, and enhancing the overall health of the carotid arteries.

Nitric Oxide Donors:

Nitric oxide, a key regulator of vascular tone and function, is the focus of pharmacological strategies involving nitric oxide donors. These agents aim to augment nitric oxide levels, promoting vasodilation and mitigating the adverse effects of endothelial dysfunction in carotid artery disease.

Personalized and Precision Medicine Approaches:

Advances in pharmacogenomics and precision medicine are paving the way for personalized treatment strategies in carotid artery disease. Tailoring pharmacological interventions based on individual genetic profiles and disease characteristics allows for more effective and targeted therapy, minimizing adverse effects and optimizing outcomes.

Conclusion:

The landscape of pharmacotherapy for carotid artery disease is undergoing a transformative phase with the emergence of novel agents targeting platelet function, inflammation, lipid metabolism, and thrombosis. These advancements hold the potential to refine current treatment strategies and improve outcomes for individuals at risk of carotid artery-related complications.

As research continues to unravel the intricate pathophysiology of carotid artery disease, the translation of these insights into innovative pharmacological therapies remains a dynamic area of investigation. The ultimate goal is to tailor interventions to individual patient needs, providing safer and more effective options for preventing stroke and optimizing vascular health in the context of carotid artery disease.

Gene Therapy in Carotid Artery Disease

Gene therapy, a revolutionary field in medical science, holds promise for addressing various cardiovascular diseases, including carotid artery disease. Carotid artery disease, characterized by atherosclerotic plaque formation in the carotid arteries, poses a substantial risk for stroke and other vascular events. In recent years, researchers have explored the potential of gene therapy as an innovative approach to modulate the underlying molecular and cellular processes associated with carotid artery disease. This section explores the current state of gene therapy research in the context of carotid artery disease.

Rationale for Gene Therapy in Carotid Artery Disease:

Targeting Atherosclerosis Pathways:

Atherosclerosis, the hallmark of carotid artery disease, involves the gradual build-up of plaques within the arterial walls. Gene therapy aims to intervene at the molecular level, targeting specific pathways involved in the initiation and progression of atherosclerosis. By modulating gene expression, researchers seek to mitigate inflammation, promote plaque stability, and reduce the overall burden of atherosclerotic lesions in the carotid arteries.

Endothelial Function Enhancement:

Preserving and enhancing endothelial function is a key aspect of gene therapy for carotid artery disease. Genes associated with endothelial nitric oxide synthase (eNOS) and nitric oxide production are of particular interest. By promoting vasodilation and reducing inflammation, gene therapies aim to improve overall vascular health and counteract endothelial dysfunction, a common feature in atherosclerosis.

Gene Therapy Approaches:

Anti-Inflammatory Genes:

Gene therapy strategies include the delivery of genes encoding anti-inflammatory proteins to counteract the chronic inflammation associated with atherosclerosis. Targeting cytokines, chemokines, and adhesion molecules involved in immune cell recruitment may help modulate the inflammatory response within the carotid arterial walls.

Plaque Stabilization Genes:

Genes associated with plaque stability, such as those involved in extracellular matrix remodeling and fibrous cap formation, are potential candidates for gene therapy. Reinforcing the fibrous cap and reducing plaque vulnerability may contribute to a more stable atherosclerotic phenotype, less prone to rupture and thrombosis.

Lipid Metabolism Genes:

Gene therapy can target lipid metabolism by regulating genes involved in cholesterol homeostasis and lipoprotein processing. Modulating the expression of genes related to LDL receptor function, cholesterol efflux, and lipoprotein lipase activity may influence the development and regression of atherosclerotic plaques.

Endothelial Nitric Oxide Synthase (eNOS) Genes:

Enhancing endothelial function through the delivery of genes associated with eNOS and nitric oxide production is a central theme in gene therapy for carotid artery disease. Augmenting nitric oxide levels promotes vasodilation, inhibits platelet aggregation, and mitigates endothelial dysfunction.

Delivery Systems:

Viral Vectors:

Viral vectors, such as adeno-associated viruses (AAVs) and lentiviruses, are commonly employed as delivery systems for gene therapy. These vectors efficiently transport therapeutic genes into target cells, facilitating their integration into the cellular genome. AAVs, in particular, are favored for their safety profile and ability to mediate long-term gene expression.

Non-Viral Vectors:

Non-viral vectors, including liposomes, nanoparticles, and electroporation techniques, offer alternative delivery methods for gene therapy. Non-viral approaches aim to overcome some limitations associated with viral vectors, such as immunogenicity and size constraints, while providing flexibility in design and administration.

Challenges and Considerations:

Immunogenicity and Safety:

The potential immunogenicity of viral vectors and the safety of long-term gene expression remain key considerations in gene therapy. Researchers are actively addressing these challenges through vector engineering, immune modulation strategies, and rigorous safety assessments in preclinical and clinical studies.

Specificity and Targeting:

Achieving precise targeting and specificity in delivering therapeutic genes to affected areas of the carotid arteries is crucial. Advances in vector design, imaging technologies, and molecular targeting strategies aim to enhance the specificity of gene delivery, minimizing off-target effects.

Preclinical and Clinical Trials:

Preclinical Studies:

Numerous preclinical studies have demonstrated the feasibility and efficacy of gene therapy in animal models of carotid artery disease. These studies provide valuable insights into the potential benefits and safety profiles of different gene therapy approaches.

Clinical Trials:

The translation of gene therapy from preclinical models to human applications is underway, with several clinical trials exploring the safety and efficacy of gene-based interventions for carotid artery disease. These trials aim to assess the feasibility of gene therapy, its impact on disease progression, and potential benefits for patients.

Future Directions:

The field of gene therapy for carotid artery disease is evolving rapidly, with ongoing research focusing on refining delivery systems, enhancing gene specificity, and addressing safety concerns. Future directions include the exploration of combinatorial gene therapies, personalized treatment approaches based on individual genetic profiles, and the integration of gene therapy into comprehensive management strategies for vascular diseases.

Conclusion:

Gene therapy represents a cutting-edge approach in the pursuit of innovative treatments for carotid artery disease. While challenges and considerations persist, the progress made in preclinical studies and the initiation of clinical trials underscore the potential of gene therapy to revolutionize the management of carotid artery disease. As research continues to unravel the intricacies of molecular and cellular pathways involved in atherosclerosis, gene therapy holds the promise of providing targeted and personalized interventions to mitigate the impact of this prevalent vascular condition.

Stem Cell Therapy in Carotid Artery Disease

Stem cell therapy has emerged as a promising avenue in regenerative medicine, offering potential solutions for various cardiovascular disorders, including carotid artery disease. Carotid artery disease, characterized by the build-up of atherosclerotic plaques in the carotid arteries, poses a significant risk for stroke and other vascular events. Stem cell therapy aims to harness the reparative and regenerative capabilities of stem cells to address the underlying pathophysiology and promote vascular health. This section explores the current state of stem cell therapy research in the context of carotid artery disease.

Rationale for Stem Cell Therapy in Carotid Artery Disease:

Vascular Repair and Regeneration:

The unique ability of stem cells to differentiate into various cell types, including vascular cells, forms the basis for their application in carotid artery disease. Stem cell therapy seeks to harness the regenerative potential of these cells to repair damaged endothelium, promote neovascularization, and contribute to the stabilization of atherosclerotic plaques.

Immunomodulation and Anti-Inflammatory Effects:

Stem cells possess immunomodulatory properties that can influence the inflammatory microenvironment associated with atherosclerosis. By modulating immune responses, stem cells may contribute to plaque stabilization and mitigate the chronic inflammation that accelerates disease progression.

Types of Stem Cells Used in Carotid Artery Disease:

Mesenchymal Stem Cells (MSCs):

MSCs, derived from various sources such as bone marrow, adipose tissue, and umbilical cord blood, are a commonly studied type of stem cell in carotid artery disease. MSCs exhibit multilineage differentiation potential and secrete factors that promote tissue repair, making them suitable candidates for vascular regeneration.

Endothelial Progenitor Cells (EPCs):

EPCs are a specific subset of stem cells with a commitment to endothelial cell lineage. These cells contribute to endothelial repair and neovascularization. Research explores the potential of EPCs to enhance endothelial function and address endothelial dysfunction in carotid artery disease.

Induced Pluripotent Stem Cells (iPSCs):

iPSCs, reprogrammed from somatic cells, have the capacity to differentiate into various cell types. Their potential in regenerative medicine is being investigated, and studies explore their application in vascular repair for conditions like carotid artery disease.

Mechanisms of Action:

Differentiation and Integration:

Stem cells can differentiate into endothelial cells, smooth muscle cells, and other cell types integral to vascular structure and function. When introduced into the diseased carotid arteries, stem cells aim to integrate into the vascular tissue, contributing to repair and regeneration.

Paracrine Effects:

The paracrine effects of stem cells involve the secretion of growth factors, cytokines, and extracellular vesicles. These factors create a regenerative microenvironment, modulate inflammation, and promote the survival and function of existing cells within the carotid arteries.

Delivery Methods:

Local Injection:

Direct injection of stem cells into the affected carotid arteries is a common delivery method. This approach allows for targeted delivery of stem cells to the site of pathology, facilitating their integration into the vascular tissue.

Systemic Infusion:

Systemic infusion involves introducing stem cells into the bloodstream, allowing them to home to the damaged areas of the carotid arteries. While less targeted than local injection, systemic infusion offers a minimally invasive approach with potential systemic benefits.

Tissue Engineering:

Advancements in tissue engineering techniques involve the creation of scaffolds or patches loaded with stem cells. These engineered tissues can be implanted in the carotid arteries to provide structural support and promote localized regeneration.

Preclinical and Clinical Studies:

Preclinical Efficacy:

Numerous preclinical studies in animal models of carotid artery disease have demonstrated the potential efficacy of stem cell therapy. These studies have shown improvements in vascular structure, endothelial function, and plaque stability following stem cell interventions.

Clinical Trials:

Clinical trials are underway to evaluate the safety and efficacy of stem cell therapy in patients with carotid artery disease. These trials aim to assess the impact of stem cell interventions on clinical outcomes, vascular function, and the progression of atherosclerosis in human subjects.

Challenges and Considerations:

Optimal Cell Type Selection:

Determining the most appropriate type of stem cell for carotid artery disease remains a critical consideration. The choice between MSCs, EPCs, or iPSCs depends on factors such as their differentiation potential, safety profile, and ease of isolation.

Immunogenicity and Allogenic Transplants:

The immunogenicity of allogeneic stem cell transplants is a potential concern. Research explores strategies to mitigate immune responses and enhance the compatibility of stem cell therapies, including the use of autologous cells or immunomodulatory approaches.

Future Directions:

The field of stem cell therapy for carotid artery disease is dynamic, with ongoing research aiming to refine therapeutic approaches, enhance delivery methods, and address current challenges. Future directions include the exploration of combination therapies, optimization of dosing regimens, and the integration of stem cell therapy into comprehensive management strategies for vascular diseases.

Conclusion:

Stem cell therapy holds significant promise as a novel approach to addressing carotid artery disease by promoting vascular repair, modulating inflammation, and contributing to overall vascular health. While challenges and considerations persist, the advancements in preclinical studies and the initiation of clinical trials underscore the potential of stem cell therapy to revolutionize the management of carotid artery disease, offering a regenerative perspective in the quest for innovative treatments.

CHAPTER 10: POST-TREATMENT CARE AND FOLLOW-UP

Monitoring and Surveillance in Carotid Artery Disease

Monitoring and surveillance play a pivotal role in the comprehensive management of carotid artery disease, providing clinicians with essential information for risk stratification, treatment decision-making, and the prevention of adverse vascular events. This section explores the various aspects of monitoring and surveillance strategies employed in the context of carotid artery disease.

Imaging Modalities:

Carotid Ultrasound:

Carotid ultrasound is a cornerstone in the monitoring of carotid artery disease. This non-invasive imaging modality allows for the assessment of plaque morphology, degree of stenosis, and the presence of hemodynamically significant lesions. Periodic carotid ultrasound examinations aid in tracking disease progression or regression, guiding therapeutic decisions, and identifying individuals at heightened risk for stroke.

Doppler Ultrasound:

Doppler ultrasound provides valuable hemodynamic information by assessing blood flow velocity within the carotid arteries. This aids in the identification of turbulent flow associated with stenotic lesions, helping to quantify the degree of stenosis and assess the risk of embolization. Doppler ultrasound complements structural imaging, offering a comprehensive evaluation of carotid artery health.

Magnetic Resonance Angiography (MRA):

Magnetic resonance angiography is a non-invasive imaging technique that utilizes magnetic fields and radio waves to generate detailed images of the carotid arteries. MRA provides high-resolution anatomical information, aiding in the visualization of plaque characteristics, luminal narrowing, and potential complications such as intraplaque hemorrhage. It is particularly useful for individuals with contraindications to contrast media.

Computed Tomography Angiography (CTA):

Computed tomography angiography involves the use of X-rays and computerized processing to create detailed images of the carotid arteries. CTA is valuable for visualizing calcified plaques, assessing the degree of stenosis, and identifying anatomical variations. It is commonly employed in the preoperative evaluation and surveillance of carotid artery disease.

Surveillance Frequency:

Asymptomatic Carotid Artery Stenosis:

For individuals with asymptomatic carotid artery stenosis, surveillance frequency is typically determined based on the severity of stenosis:

- Mild Stenosis (0-29%): Surveillance may be recommended every 3 to 5 years.
- Moderate Stenosis (30-69%): Surveillance intervals may be shortened to every 1 to 2 years.
- Severe Stenosis (70% or more): Close monitoring, with intervals as short as every 6 months, is often advised.

Symptomatic Carotid Artery Disease:

In cases of symptomatic carotid artery disease, where individuals have experienced transient ischemic attacks (TIAs) or strokes related to carotid artery stenosis, more frequent surveillance is typically warranted. The frequency of monitoring may be determined by the severity of stenosis, the response to therapeutic interventions, and the overall risk profile of the patient.

Functional Assessments:

1 Transcranial Doppler (TCD):

Transcranial Doppler ultrasound assesses blood flow in the intracranial arteries. It is employed to monitor cerebral hemodynamics, detect microemboli, and assess collateral circulation. TCD can provide valuable insights into the risk of embolic events and guide treatment decisions in individuals with carotid artery disease.

Cerebral Perfusion Imaging:

Functional imaging techniques, such as single-photon emission computed tomography (SPECT) or positron emission tomography (PET), can assess cerebral perfusion. These modalities aid in evaluating the impact of carotid artery disease on cerebral blood flow and identifying areas of compromised perfusion, particularly in individuals with complex or symptomatic disease.

Risk Factor Monitoring:

In addition to imaging and functional assessments, ongoing monitoring of modifiable risk factors is integral to the management of carotid artery disease:

Blood Pressure Control:

Regular monitoring of blood pressure is essential to manage hypertension, a significant risk factor for carotid artery disease. Tight blood pressure control is crucial for reducing the progression of atherosclerosis and minimizing the risk of vascular events.

Lipid Profile:

Periodic assessment of lipid levels guides the management of dyslipidemia, another modifiable risk factor. Targeted lipid-lowering therapies aim to maintain optimal cholesterol levels, slowing the progression of atherosclerosis and reducing the risk of plaque rupture.

Diabetes Management:

For individuals with diabetes, regular monitoring of blood glucose levels is imperative. Optimal glycemic control is essential for mitigating the impact of diabetes on vascular health and preventing accelerated atherosclerosis.

Response to Interventions:

For individuals undergoing interventions such as carotid endarterectomy (CEA) or carotid artery stenting (CAS), post-procedural monitoring is crucial:

Ultrasound Surveillance:

Regular post-procedural ultrasound assessments monitor the patency of the treated carotid artery, assess for restenosis, and ensure the effectiveness of the intervention. The frequency of surveillance may vary based on the type of intervention and individual patient characteristics.

Neurological Assessment:

Close neurological monitoring is essential to detect any post-interventional complications, such as stroke or transient neurological deficits. Regular assessments aid in the early identification of adverse events and prompt intervention if necessary.

Patient Education and Lifestyle Monitoring:

Empowering patients with knowledge about their condition and promoting healthy lifestyle choices are integral components of monitoring and surveillance:

Lifestyle Counseling:

Regular counseling on lifestyle modifications, including smoking cessation, dietary changes, and physical activity, contributes to long-term vascular health. Monitoring patient adherence to these recommendations is an ongoing process.

Medication Adherence:

Ensuring patients adhere to prescribed medications, including antiplatelet agents, lipid-lowering drugs, and antihypertensive medications, is vital. Monitoring medication adherence contributes to the overall management of cardiovascular risk factors.

Multidisciplinary Approach:

A multidisciplinary approach involving collaboration between vascular specialists, neurologists, radiologists, and primary care physicians enhances the effectiveness of monitoring and surveillance. Regular interdisciplinary discussions facilitate comprehensive assessments and informed decision-making based on the evolving clinical picture of carotid artery disease.

Conclusion:

Monitoring and surveillance are integral components of the holistic management of carotid artery disease, providing a dynamic framework for risk assessment, treatment planning, and ongoing patient care. The judicious selection of imaging modalities, functional assessments, and risk factor monitoring, coupled with patient education and a multidisciplinary approach, ensures a comprehensive and personalized approach to the management of individuals with carotid artery disease. Regular surveillance not only aids in the early detection of complications but also empowers individuals to actively participate in their vascular health, contributing to improved long-term outcomes.

Rehabilitation and Lifestyle Modification in Carotid Artery Disease

Rehabilitation and lifestyle modification are integral components of the comprehensive management strategy for individuals with carotid artery disease. These interventions aim to optimize vascular health, reduce cardiovascular risk factors, and improve overall well-being. This section explores the key aspects of rehabilitation and lifestyle modification in the context of carotid artery disease.

Cardiac Rehabilitation:

Exercise Training:

Structured exercise programs form the cornerstone of cardiac rehabilitation for individuals with carotid artery disease.

Aerobic exercise, such as walking, cycling, and swimming, promotes cardiovascular fitness, enhances endothelial function, and contributes to overall cardiovascular health. Exercise prescriptions are tailored to individual capacities, ensuring safety and adherence.

Resistance Training:

Incorporating resistance training into rehabilitation programs helps strengthen muscles and improve overall functional capacity. Resistance exercises may include weightlifting, resistance bands, or bodyweight exercises, with careful consideration of individual fitness levels and medical history.

Supervised Sessions:

Supervised cardiac rehabilitation sessions, conducted by trained healthcare professionals, offer a supportive environment for individuals with carotid artery disease. Regular monitoring of vital signs, exercise intensity, and overall well-being ensures a safe and effective rehabilitation experience.

Lifestyle Modification:

Smoking Cessation:

Smoking is a major modifiable risk factor for carotid artery disease. Smoking cessation programs, including counseling and pharmacotherapy, support individuals in breaking the habit. Quitting smoking not only reduces the risk of disease progression but also contributes to overall cardiovascular health.

Dietary Changes:

Nutritional interventions focus on heart-healthy dietary patterns, emphasizing:

- **Mediterranean Diet:** Rich in fruits, vegetables, whole

grains, and healthy fats, the Mediterranean diet is associated with reduced cardiovascular risk. It emphasizes lean proteins, nuts, and olive oil while limiting saturated fats and processed foods.
- **DASH Diet:** The Dietary Approaches to Stop Hypertension (DASH) diet emphasizes a low-sodium, high-potassium, and nutrient-rich eating plan, beneficial for managing hypertension, a common risk factor for carotid artery disease.
- **Low-Fat, Low-Cholesterol Diet:** Restricting dietary sources of saturated and trans fats helps manage cholesterol levels, supporting the prevention of atherosclerosis.

Weight Management:

Maintaining a healthy weight is crucial for individuals with carotid artery disease. Lifestyle modifications, including portion control, regular physical activity, and dietary adjustments, contribute to weight management and reduce the burden of cardiovascular risk factors.

Blood Pressure Control:

Adopting lifestyle measures to control blood pressure includes:

- **Reducing Sodium Intake:** Limiting salt in the diet helps manage hypertension.
- **Regular Physical Activity:** Engaging in regular exercise contributes to blood pressure regulation.
- **Stress Management:** Techniques such as meditation, deep breathing, and mindfulness aid in stress reduction, positively impacting blood pressure.

Diabetes Management:

For individuals with diabetes, effective management of blood glucose levels is paramount. Lifestyle modifications, including a balanced diet, regular exercise, and medication adherence, contribute to glycemic control and reduce the risk of vascular complications.

Psychological Support:

Stress Management:

Chronic stress can adversely impact cardiovascular health. Stress management techniques, such as mindfulness, relaxation exercises, and counseling, help individuals cope with stressors and promote emotional well-being.

Mental Health Support:

Addressing mental health concerns, including anxiety and depression, is crucial in the overall management of carotid artery disease. Collaborative care involving mental health professionals contributes to holistic patient care.

Medication Adherence:

Ensuring adherence to prescribed medications is essential for managing cardiovascular risk factors. Healthcare providers work collaboratively with patients to educate them about the importance of medications, address concerns, and monitor for any adverse effects.

Education and Empowerment:

Empowering individuals with knowledge about their condition, risk factors, and the importance of lifestyle modifications is fundamental:

Patient Education Programs:

Structured educational programs provide information about carotid artery disease, its management, and lifestyle interventions. These programs empower individuals to make informed decisions about their health and actively participate in their care.

Individualized Goal Setting:

Setting achievable and individualized goals, whether related to exercise, dietary changes, or smoking cessation, enhances motivation and promotes sustained lifestyle modifications. Collaborative goal-setting between healthcare providers and patients ensures realistic and meaningful outcomes.

Long-Term Follow-Up:

Long-term follow-up involves ongoing monitoring of lifestyle habits, cardiovascular risk factors, and overall well-being. Regular assessments enable healthcare providers to adjust interventions, address emerging concerns, and reinforce positive lifestyle choices.

Conclusion:

Rehabilitation and lifestyle modification are essential components of the holistic management of carotid artery disease. By incorporating structured exercise, promoting healthy lifestyle choices, and addressing psychological well-being, these interventions contribute to the overall cardiovascular health of individuals. Empowering patients through education and ongoing support ensures sustained adherence to lifestyle modifications, fostering long-term vascular health and reducing the risk of adverse cardiovascular events. The integration of rehabilitation and lifestyle modification into the comprehensive care plan exemplifies a patient-centered approach, emphasizing the importance of holistic well-being in the management of carotid artery disease.

Long-Term Outcomes and Recurrence in Carotid Artery Disease

Understanding the long-term outcomes and the potential for recurrence is crucial in the comprehensive management of carotid artery disease. This section explores the trajectory of the disease over time, the impact of interventions, and strategies to mitigate the risk of recurrence.

Natural History of Carotid Artery Disease:

Progression of Atherosclerosis:

Carotid artery disease, primarily driven by atherosclerosis, exhibits a variable progression over time. Factors such as age, genetic predisposition, and the presence of modifiable risk factors influence the natural history of atherosclerotic plaques within the carotid arteries. Understanding this progression is crucial for risk stratification and determining the appropriate intensity of monitoring and intervention.

Complications and Sequelae:

The natural history of carotid artery disease may lead to various complications, including plaque rupture, thrombosis, and embolization. These events can result in transient ischemic attacks (TIAs), strokes, or other vascular incidents. Monitoring for complications and their potential impact on long-term outcomes is essential for timely intervention.

Post-Intervention Outcomes:

Carotid Endarterectomy (CEA):

Long-term outcomes following carotid endarterectomy (CEA) are generally favorable, with a significant reduction in the risk of stroke for individuals with symptomatic and high-grade asymptomatic carotid artery stenosis. Regular surveillance is crucial to detect restenosis or other complications that may impact long-term outcomes.

Carotid Artery Stenting (CAS):

Carotid artery stenting (CAS) has demonstrated effectiveness in certain populations, offering an alternative to CEA. Long-term outcomes following CAS require careful monitoring for restenosis, procedural complications, and the prevention of recurrent vascular events.

Risk of Recurrence:

Factors Influencing Recurrence:

Several factors contribute to the risk of recurrence in carotid artery disease:

- **Degree of Stenosis:** Higher degrees of stenosis increase the risk of recurrent vascular events.
- **Presence of Symptoms:** Individuals with symptomatic carotid artery disease are at a higher risk of recurrence compared to those with asymptomatic disease.
- **Coexisting Cardiovascular Risk Factors:** Uncontrolled hypertension, diabetes, smoking, and dyslipidemia contribute to an elevated risk of recurrence.
- **Plaque Characteristics:** Vulnerable plaques with features like thin fibrous caps and large lipid cores are associated with an increased risk of rupture and recurrence.

Importance of Ongoing Surveillance:

Regular surveillance, including imaging studies and clinical assessments, is essential for identifying recurrent disease or new vascular events. Surveillance allows for prompt intervention and adjustments to the management plan based on the evolving clinical picture.

Secondary Prevention Strategies:

Medications for Secondary Prevention:

The use of medications plays a crucial role in secondary prevention:

- **Antiplatelet Agents:** Aspirin or other antiplatelet agents are commonly prescribed to reduce the risk of thrombotic events.
- **Lipid-Lowering Drugs:** Statins and other lipid-lowering medications manage dyslipidemia, contributing to plaque stabilization and reduced cardiovascular risk.
- **Antihypertensive Medications:** Blood pressure control is paramount in preventing recurrence, and antihypertensive medications are tailored to individual needs.

Lifestyle Modification:

Continued adherence to lifestyle modifications is integral to long-term success:

- **Healthy Diet:** Maintaining a heart-healthy diet, such as the Mediterranean or DASH diet, supports overall cardiovascular health.
- **Regular Exercise:** Ongoing physical activity contributes to fitness, weight management, and the prevention of modifiable risk factors.
- **Smoking Cessation:** Continued efforts to quit smoking or maintain abstinence are crucial for reducing recurrence risk.

Education and Empowerment:

Empowering individuals with knowledge about their condition, the importance of medications, and the role of lifestyle modifications fosters active participation in their care. Regular follow-up visits provide opportunities for education, goal-setting, and addressing any concerns or challenges.

Multidisciplinary Approach:

A multidisciplinary approach involving vascular specialists, neurologists, primary care physicians, and other healthcare professionals ensures comprehensive and coordinated care. Regular case discussions, shared decision-making, and a unified approach contribute to optimal long-term outcomes.

Patient Counseling and Quality of Life:

Addressing Patient Concerns:

Effective communication with patients regarding their prognosis, ongoing management, and potential complications is essential. Addressing concerns and providing realistic expectations contribute to patient confidence and engagement in long-term care.

Quality of Life Considerations:

Long-term outcomes extend beyond clinical parameters to include the quality of life for individuals with carotid artery disease. Assessing and addressing factors such as psychological well-being, functional status, and social support contribute to an improved overall quality of life.

Future Directions in Long-Term Management:

Ongoing research aims to refine long-term management strategies, exploring novel interventions, optimizing surveillance techniques, and personalizing care based on individual characteristics. Advancements in understanding the molecular and genetic basis of carotid artery disease may pave the way for targeted therapies and precision medicine approaches.

Conclusion:

Long-term outcomes and the risk of recurrence in carotid artery disease are influenced by a complex interplay of factors. Regular surveillance, secondary prevention strategies, and ongoing multidisciplinary care are integral to optimizing outcomes and enhancing the quality of life for individuals affected by this vascular condition. As research progresses, the refinement of management strategies and the integration of innovative approaches will contribute to further improving long-term outcomes in carotid artery disease.

CHAPTER 11: INTEGRATIVE AND HOLISTIC APPROACHES

Role of Nutrition and Supplements in Carotid Artery Disease

Nutrition plays a pivotal role in the management of carotid artery disease, influencing the progression of atherosclerosis, modulation of risk factors, and overall cardiovascular health. This section explores the significance of dietary choices and the potential role of supplements in supporting individuals with carotid artery disease.

Heart-Healthy Dietary Patterns:

Mediterranean Diet:

The Mediterranean diet, characterized by high consumption of fruits, vegetables, whole grains, nuts, and olive oil, is associated with cardiovascular benefits. Rich in antioxidants, fiber, and monounsaturated fats, this dietary pattern may contribute to reduced inflammation, improved lipid profiles, and overall vascular health.

DASH Diet:

The Dietary Approaches to Stop Hypertension (DASH) diet emphasizes the consumption of fruits, vegetables, low-fat dairy, lean proteins, and whole grains while limiting sodium intake. DASH is designed to manage blood pressure, a critical factor in the progression of carotid artery disease.

Low-Fat, Low-Cholesterol Diet:

Reducing dietary intake of saturated and trans fats is essential for managing cholesterol levels. This dietary approach, coupled with increased consumption of heart-healthy fats, supports the prevention of atherosclerosis and plaque formation.

Key Nutrients and Supplements:

Omega-3 Fatty Acids:

Omega-3 fatty acids, found in fatty fish (e.g., salmon, mackerel, and sardines), flaxseeds, and walnuts, possess anti-inflammatory properties and may contribute to cardiovascular health. Omega-3 supplements, particularly EPA and DHA, may be considered in consultation with healthcare providers to support lipid management.

Antioxidants:

Antioxidants, found in fruits and vegetables, help combat oxidative stress and inflammation. Vitamins C and E, along with flavonoids and polyphenols, may contribute to the maintenance of vascular health. However, obtaining antioxidants through whole foods is preferred over supplementation.

Vitamin D:

Vitamin D, obtained from sunlight exposure and certain foods (e.g., fatty fish, fortified dairy products), is crucial for bone health and may have cardiovascular implications. Vitamin D supplementation is recommended when there is deficiency, but its specific role in carotid artery disease requires further research.

Coenzyme Q10 (CoQ10):

CoQ10, present in some foods and available as a supplement, is involved in cellular energy production. While studies on its efficacy in cardiovascular health are inconclusive, CoQ10 supplementation may be considered in consultation with healthcare providers.

Folate and B Vitamins:

Folate and B vitamins play a role in homocysteine metabolism. Elevated homocysteine levels are associated with increased cardiovascular risk. While supplementation with B vitamins may be considered for individuals with hyperhomocysteinemia, obtaining these nutrients from a balanced diet is preferred.

Dietary Sodium Management:

Sodium Restriction:

Reducing dietary sodium intake is crucial for managing blood pressure. Individuals with carotid artery disease are advised to limit the consumption of high-sodium foods, such as processed and packaged items. Emphasizing fresh, whole foods and using herbs and spices for flavoring supports a low-sodium diet.

Individualized Nutritional Counseling:

Personalized Dietary Plans:

Nutritional counseling tailored to individual needs, preferences, and health status is essential. Registered dietitians collaborate with individuals to develop realistic and sustainable dietary plans that address specific risk factors, including hypertension, dyslipidemia, and diabetes.

Caloric Intake and Weight Management:

Maintaining a healthy weight is integral to managing cardiovascular risk factors. Individualized nutritional counseling addresses caloric needs, promotes portion control, and supports weight management through a balanced and nutrient-dense diet.

Considerations for Nutritional Supplements:

Consultation with Healthcare Providers:

Before initiating any nutritional supplements, individuals with carotid artery disease should consult their healthcare providers. Personalized advice ensures that supplements align with individual health goals, medical conditions, and potential interactions with medications.

Monitoring for Interactions:

Certain supplements may interact with medications commonly prescribed in carotid artery disease management. Monitoring for potential interactions, especially with anticoagulants and antiplatelet agents, is crucial to avoid adverse effects.

Lifestyle Integration:

Holistic Health Approach:

Nutrition is an integral component of a holistic approach to health. Lifestyle modifications, including dietary choices, regular physical activity, and stress management, collectively contribute to cardiovascular well-being.

Ongoing Research and Emerging Insights:

Exploration of Novel Nutritional Approaches:

Ongoing research explores novel nutritional approaches, including the impact of specific food components, dietary patterns, and personalized nutrition on carotid artery disease. Emerging insights may provide additional strategies for optimizing nutritional interventions.

Conclusion:

Nutrition plays a crucial role in the management of carotid artery disease, influencing atherosclerosis, risk factors, and overall cardiovascular health. Embracing heart-healthy dietary patterns, obtaining key nutrients from whole foods, and considering supplements under guidance contribute to a comprehensive approach. Individualized nutritional counseling, lifestyle integration, and ongoing research underscore the dynamic nature of nutrition in supporting individuals with carotid artery disease on their journey towards cardiovascular health.

Mind-Body Practices in Carotid Artery Disease Management

Mind-body practices encompass a diverse range of techniques that integrate mental, emotional, and physical well-being. In the context of carotid artery disease management, these practices play a valuable role in reducing stress, improving overall mental health, and potentially influencing cardiovascular outcomes. This section explores various mind-body practices and their potential benefits in individuals with carotid artery disease.

Meditation:

Mindfulness Meditation:

Mindfulness meditation involves cultivating awareness of the present moment, fostering a non-judgmental and accepting mindset. Regular practice may contribute to stress reduction, improved emotional regulation, and enhanced overall well-being. Individuals with carotid artery disease can benefit from mindfulness meditation to manage the psychological impact of their condition.

Transcendental Meditation (TM):

Transcendental Meditation is a specific form of mantra meditation associated with a state of deep restful awareness. Research suggests potential benefits for blood pressure reduction and stress management. While more studies are needed in the context of carotid artery disease, TM offers a non-invasive approach to support cardiovascular health.

Yoga:

Hatha Yoga:

Hatha Yoga combines physical postures (asanas), breath control (pranayama), and meditation to promote flexibility, balance, and relaxation. Regular practice may contribute to stress reduction, improved cardiovascular function, and enhanced quality of life for individuals with carotid artery disease.

Restorative Yoga:

Restorative yoga emphasizes relaxation and stress relief through gentle poses and deep breathing. This form of yoga is particularly beneficial for individuals with carotid artery disease, providing a soothing practice that can be adapted to various fitness levels.

Tai Chi:

Tai Chi is a mind-body practice originating from traditional Chinese martial arts. Characterized by slow, flowing movements and focused breath control, Tai Chi promotes balance, flexibility, and relaxation. Preliminary research suggests potential benefits for blood pressure control and stress reduction, making it a suitable option for individuals with carotid artery disease.

Biofeedback:

Biofeedback involves using electronic monitoring to provide individuals with real-time information about physiological processes such as heart rate, muscle tension, and skin temperature. Learning to control these processes through feedback may help individuals manage stress and potentially influence cardiovascular health. While more research is needed, biofeedback holds promise as an adjunctive therapy in carotid artery disease management.

Guided Imagery:

Guided imagery involves using mental images to promote relaxation and alleviate stress. Individuals with carotid artery disease can benefit from guided imagery sessions that focus on positive visualizations, fostering a sense of calmness and well-being. This practice may contribute to overall stress reduction and improved mental health.

Breathing Exercises:

Diaphragmatic Breathing:

Diaphragmatic breathing, or deep abdominal breathing, involves consciously engaging the diaphragm to promote slower and deeper breaths. This technique can activate the body's relaxation response, reducing stress and potentially influencing blood pressure regulation.

Resonant Breathing:

Resonant breathing involves breathing at a specific rate to optimize heart rate variability, a marker of autonomic nervous system balance. This practice may contribute to stress reduction and cardiovascular health. Individuals with carotid artery disease can incorporate resonant breathing into their routine under guidance.

Progressive Muscle Relaxation (PMR):

PMR involves systematically tensing and then relaxing different muscle groups to promote physical and mental relaxation. Regular practice can help individuals with carotid artery disease manage stress, reduce muscle tension, and improve overall well-being.

Integrative Mind-Body Programs:

Integrative mind-body programs, such as Mind-Body Medicine and Mindfulness-Based Stress Reduction (MBSR), offer comprehensive approaches to stress reduction and well-being. These programs often include a combination of meditation, yoga, and other mind-body practices. While research in the context of carotid artery disease is limited, these holistic programs may contribute to improved mental health and resilience.

Considerations for Implementation:

Individualized Approaches:

Mind-body practices should be tailored to individual preferences, capabilities, and health conditions. Healthcare providers can collaborate with individuals to identify practices that align with their needs and goals.

Safety Precautions:

Individuals with carotid artery disease should consult their healthcare providers before initiating any new mind-body practice, especially if they have coexisting health conditions or concerns. Safety considerations and modifications can be discussed to ensure a positive and safe experience.

Potential Benefits:

Stress Reduction:

Mind-body practices contribute to stress reduction by promoting relaxation, fostering a positive mindset, and enhancing emotional well-being. Chronic stress is a modifiable risk factor that may influence the progression of carotid artery disease.

Blood Pressure Management:

Some mind-body practices, such as meditation and deep breathing, have shown potential benefits for blood pressure management. While not a replacement for medical interventions, these practices may complement standard care.

Quality of Life Improvement:

Engaging in mind-body practices has the potential to improve overall quality of life for individuals with carotid artery disease. By addressing psychological well-being, these practices contribute to a holistic approach to health.

Integration into Comprehensive Care:

Mind-body practices should be integrated into a comprehensive care plan for individuals with carotid artery disease. Collaboration between healthcare providers, including cardiologists, neurologists, and mental health professionals, ensures a cohesive approach to addressing both physical and mental aspects of health.

Conclusion:

Mind-body practices offer a holistic approach to carotid artery disease management, focusing on the interconnectedness of mental and physical well-being. By incorporating meditation, yoga, breathing exercises, and other techniques, individuals with carotid artery disease can potentially reduce stress, improve cardiovascular health, and enhance their overall quality of life. As part of a comprehensive care plan, mind-body practices contribute to a patient-centered approach that considers the multifaceted nature of health and well-being.

Exercise and Physical Activity in Carotid Artery Disease Management

Exercise and physical activity are integral components of the comprehensive management of carotid artery disease. Regular physical activity not only contributes to overall cardiovascular health but also plays a crucial role in reducing risk factors associated with the progression of atherosclerosis. This section explores the benefits of exercise, types of physical activity, and considerations for individuals with carotid artery disease.

Benefits of Exercise:

Cardiovascular Fitness:

Regular exercise improves cardiovascular fitness by enhancing the efficiency of the heart and lungs. Improved aerobic capacity contributes to better circulation, oxygen delivery, and overall cardiovascular function.

Blood Pressure Regulation:

Physical activity helps regulate blood pressure, a critical factor in the progression of carotid artery disease. Engaging in regular exercise supports optimal blood pressure levels and may contribute to the prevention of complications.

Lipid Profile Improvement:

Exercise influences lipid metabolism, leading to favorable changes in lipid profiles. It can raise high-density lipoprotein (HDL or "good" cholesterol) and lower low-density lipoprotein (LDL or "bad" cholesterol), reducing the risk of atherosclerosis.

Weight Management:

Maintaining a healthy weight is essential for individuals with carotid artery disease. Exercise contributes to weight management by burning calories, improving metabolism, and supporting overall energy balance.

Glucose Regulation:

Regular physical activity helps regulate blood glucose levels, especially important for individuals with diabetes. Improved glucose control contributes to the management of a key cardiovascular risk factor.

Stress Reduction:

Exercise is a powerful stress-reduction tool, promoting the release of endorphins and reducing levels of stress hormones. Managing stress is crucial for individuals with carotid artery disease, as chronic stress can impact cardiovascular health.

Improved Mental Health:

Physical activity has positive effects on mental health, reducing symptoms of anxiety and depression. Maintaining mental well-being is essential for the overall quality of life of individuals with carotid artery disease.

Types of Exercise:

Aerobic Exercise:

Aerobic exercise, such as brisk walking, jogging, cycling, and swimming, is beneficial for cardiovascular health. It improves endurance, strengthens the heart, and supports overall circulation.

Resistance Training:

Resistance training involves using weights, resistance bands, or bodyweight exercises to strengthen muscles. This type of exercise is essential for overall physical fitness and may contribute to improved functional capacity.

Flexibility and Stretching:

Flexibility exercises, including stretching and yoga, enhance joint mobility and reduce the risk of injury. These exercises are particularly important for individuals with carotid artery disease to maintain overall physical function.

Balance and Stability Exercises:

Balance and stability exercises, such as Tai Chi, help improve coordination and reduce the risk of falls. These exercises are valuable for individuals with carotid artery disease, especially those at risk of complications.

Considerations for Exercise in Carotid Artery Disease:

Medical Clearance:

Before initiating an exercise program, individuals with carotid artery disease should obtain medical clearance from their healthcare providers. This ensures that exercise recommendations align with individual health status and potential limitations.

Individualized Exercise Plans:

Exercise plans should be tailored to individual preferences, fitness levels, and any existing health conditions. Collaborating with healthcare providers and, if necessary, exercise physiologists ensures the development of safe and effective exercise routines.

Gradual Progression:

For individuals with carotid artery disease, especially those new to exercise, gradual progression is essential. Starting with low-intensity activities and gradually increasing duration and intensity helps prevent overexertion and reduces the risk of complications.

Monitoring for Symptoms:

Individuals engaged in physical activity should be aware of potential symptoms, such as chest pain, shortness of breath, or dizziness. Monitoring for these symptoms allows for prompt evaluation and adjustment of exercise plans as needed.

Cardiovascular Rehabilitation:

Role of Cardiovascular Rehabilitation:

Cardiovascular rehabilitation programs are structured interventions that combine exercise, education, and support for individuals with cardiovascular conditions, including carotid artery disease. These programs, conducted under the supervision of healthcare professionals, offer a comprehensive approach to improving cardiovascular health.

Components of Cardiovascular Rehabilitation:

Cardiovascular rehabilitation typically includes:

- **Supervised Exercise Training:** Tailored exercise programs under professional supervision.
- **Education:** Information on heart-healthy living, risk factor management, and medication adherence.
- **Psychosocial Support:** Counseling and support for mental well-being.

- **Lifestyle Modification:** Guidance on dietary choices, smoking cessation, and stress management.

Benefits of Cardiovascular Rehabilitation:

Participation in cardiovascular rehabilitation has been associated with:

- **Improved Cardiovascular Fitness:** Enhanced aerobic capacity and endurance.
- **Risk Factor Reduction:** Better management of blood pressure, cholesterol, and diabetes.
- **Quality of Life Improvement:** Enhanced overall well-being and mental health.

Lifestyle Integration:

Incorporating Physical Activity into Daily Life:

Encouraging individuals with carotid artery disease to incorporate physical activity into their daily routines is essential. This may include activities such as walking, cycling, or gardening, fostering a sustainable and active lifestyle.

Collaborative Approach:

Healthcare providers, including cardiologists, physiotherapists, and exercise specialists, play a crucial role in promoting physical activity. Collaborative efforts ensure that exercise recommendations align with individual health needs and goals.

Long-Term Commitment:

Sustainable Exercise Habits:

Establishing sustainable exercise habits is crucial for long-term cardiovascular health. Individuals with carotid artery disease are encouraged to view physical activity as a lifelong commitment to maintaining overall well-being.

Periodic Reassessment:

Periodic reassessment of exercise plans ensures that they remain aligned with individual health status and goals. Adjustments can be made as needed to accommodate changes in fitness levels, preferences, or health conditions.

Future Directions in Exercise Research:

Exploring Innovative Approaches:

Ongoing research explores innovative approaches to exercise, including personalized exercise prescriptions, tele-rehabilitation, and virtual reality-based programs. These advancements aim to enhance accessibility and adherence to exercise regimens.

Adapting to Technological Advances:

Integration of wearable devices, mobile applications, and remote monitoring technologies can facilitate home-based exercise programs. Embracing technological advances enhances the flexibility and inclusivity of exercise interventions for individuals with carotid artery disease.

Conclusion:

Exercise and physical activity are cornerstones of carotid artery disease management, contributing to overall cardiovascular health, risk factor reduction, and improved quality of life. Engaging in regular aerobic, resistance, and flexibility exercises, tailored to individual needs, forms a crucial part of a comprehensive care plan. By promoting physical activity, healthcare providers empower individuals with carotid artery disease to actively participate in the optimization of their cardiovascular well-being. As research continues to unravel the benefits of exercise, the integration of innovative approaches ensures ongoing advancements in the field of exercise and physical activity in carotid artery disease management.

Printed in Great Britain
by Amazon